Unlocking the Potential Within: Müller Glia as a Key to Treating Retinal Diseases

Sheena

Table of Contents

Chapter 1

General Introduction

The retina is a thin lining of neural tissue that lines the back of the eye that is responsible for the conversion of environmental light into electrochemical signals. These signals are transmitted into the brain to enable the sense of vision. Visual senses are often regarded as the most important sensory function, and the loss of visual acuity or blindness can have a substantial impact on an individual's quality of life.

Retinal disease is the most common cause of blindness in children, and is the most common cause of irreversible adult blindness in the Western world (Common Eye Disorders | Basics | VHI | CDC; Gilbert and Foster, 2001). While most individual causes of irreversible blindness are uncommon, they collectively represent a substantial demographic of individuals around the world. There are over 25 million adults in the United States living with visual impairment leading to economic burden of over $180 billion (Scott et al., 2016; Vision impairment and blindness). The decrease in visual acuity in retinal disease is due to the loss of retinal neurons. Currently there are no therapeutics available to restore lost retinal neurons, only prophylactic treatment to delay neuronal death in diseases such as diabetic retinopathy and glaucoma. Vision research has focused on therapeutic strategies to restore neuronal populations through endogenous mechanisms of regeneration.

The focus of this book is to better understand the process of Müller glia reprogramming, to further advance the therapeutic potential of endogenous glia to neuron cell replacement strategies. Müller glia are the primary support cell of the retina and have been shown to have the capability to form neurogenic progenitor cells in

1

response to injury. However, the efficiency of reprogramming neurons from Müller glia is limited in mammalian species, and future therapeutic advancements will rely on a more comprehensive understanding of this transformative mechanism for restoring vision in sight-threatening diseases.

Overview of Retinal Anatomy

The vertebrate retina is a thin neural tissue that originates from the optic nerve, where it enters the back of the eye and radiates from the central to peripheral hemispheres of the globe. The retina is organized into distinct layers of cells, with three layers of cell bodies and residing nuclei, and two inner and outer synaptic plexiform layers (OPL, IPL). The outmost layer of the retina consists of the photoreceptors, with their outer segments resting proximally to supporting pigmented retinal epithelium and vascular choroidal layer of connective tissue. The photoreceptor layer (PRL) consists of the inner and outer segments of the rod and cone photoreceptors, and their nuclei reside in the outer nuclear layer (ONL). The inner nuclear layer (INL) consists of amacrine, bipolar, and horizontal neurons. Ganglion cells are projection neurons that reside in the ganglion cell layer (GCL), whose axons travel in the nerve fiber layer (NFL) and accumulate in the central retina to form the optic nerve.

The vertebrate retina also contains different glial subtypes that support normal retinal function. The primary glial cell is Müller glia, whose cell bodies are oriented in the INL, and extend their processes through the full thickness of the retina, with exception of the PRL. In the vascular retina of vertebrates, there are astrocytes that are associated with the vasculature and are distributed in the NFL, GCL, and IPL. Avascular retinas often lack astrocytes, but possess oligodendrocytes that myelinate ganglion cell axons in the NFL (Kohsaka et al., 1980). Some species also contain a unique cell type that does not possess classical astrocyte or oligodendrocyte markers, called nonastrocytic inner retinal glia (NIRG) (Fischer et al., 2010). Microglia, the resident immune cell of the central nervous system, has been found in the retinas of vertebrate species, typically residing predominantly in the plexiform layers and NFL.

The anatomy of the retina is important to carrying out its physiologic function of converting photons of light into electrochemical signals that are perceived as visual senses. A photon of light enters through the full thickness of the retinal tissue to activate light sensitive pigments that result in a graded change in the membrane potential (Demb and Singer, 2015). This change is propagated through vertical transmission, first to bipolar cells, then to ganglion cells. Horizontal and amacrine interneurons have lateral interactions that help to process and refine the visual signals prior transmitting the signal out of the retina (Demb and Singer, 2015). The ganglion cell axons leave the eye as the optic nerve, segregate their receptive hemisphere in the optic chiasm and synapse in the lateral geniculate nucleus, ultimately being processed in the optic lobe (Demb and Singer, 2015).

Patterning of Retinal Development

Retinal tissue possesses a strictly organized stratification possessing several neuronal types and subtypes that are necessary for visual perception. Temporally regulated retinal development is highly conserved among species (Wilson and Houart, 2004). The retinal tissue originates as with early regional "eye field" specification of the diencephalon with the upregulation of transcription factors Pax6, Six3, Six6, Tbx3, Lhx2, Rx, and T11 (Zuber et al., 2003). These multipotent cells evaginates as the optic vesicles and will proceed to form every neuronal cell type of the mature postnatal retina (Turner and Cepko, 1987). The pattern of specification is broadly categorized as early and late born neurons (Livesey and Cepko, 2001). Ganglion, horizontal and cone photoreceptors are formed first, followed by the later born rod, bipolar, and amacrine cells(Cepko, 2014). After neuronal specification, these progenitors undergo phase of gliogenesis resulting in Müller glia formation. Other glia are not formed intrinsically by the retinal progenitor cells (Cepko, 2014). The oligodendrocyte precursors and astrocytes migrate in from the optic nerve along the nerve fiber layer (Rompani and Cepko, 2010). The microglia are derived from yolk sac mesoderm and migrate into the retina during development via the optic nerve (Ginhoux et al., 2010).

Physiologic Functions of Müller glia

Müller glia are the primary glial cell of the vertebrate retina. Their cell bodies are located in the INL, and their processes span from the ONL out to the NFL. The cells occupy a large area and their multiple processes allow them to contact the diverse subtypes of the retina to facilitate support functions. Similar to astrocytes, Müller glia serve an array of supportive functions integral to the physiologic function of the retinal parenchyma (Bringmann et al., 2009). The longitudinal orientation of Müller glia spanning the retina provides structural support and reinforces the retina from shear stress and reinforces the blood-retinal barrier in a vascular retina (Reichenbach and Bringmann, 2013). They express intermediate filaments that span the cell, such as vimentin and GFAP to provide cellular stability and structure to the surrounding tissue (Reichenbach and Bringmann, 2013). Disorders of Müller glia in humans results in macular telangiectasias, which causes fragile vessel rupture of the macula to reduce central vision (Powner et al., 2013).

Müller glia interact with neuronal synapses by providing neurotransmitter recycling. Müller glia highly express glutamate aspartate transporter (GLAST), which uptakes excitatory glutamate from the synapse (Derouiche and Rauen, 1995). Müller glia also express glutamine synthetase (GS) that converts glutamate to glutamine, which is then recycled back to neurons to serve as a precursor for GABA and glutamate (Pow and Crook, 1995; Pow and Crook, 1996). Müller glia also participate in the secretion and regulation of "gliotransmitters" that modulate synaptic strength. Molecules such as ATP can sensitize ion channels to produce a larger excitatory post synaptic potential, where adenosine can have an inverse effect of dampening the receptivity of the post synaptic neuron (Newman, 2004).

Muller glia are also involved in the siphoning of extracellular potassium. The firing of action potentials from surrounding neurons results in a sodium influx and a potassium efflux. The microenvironment of rapidly firing neurons can result in the accumulation of extracellular potassium that can exceed the capacity of neuronal sodium potassium ATP pumps, which results in the slower repolarization and can hamper the frequency of neuronal firing or predispose neurons to excitotoxicity (Bringmann et al., 2006). Several potassium channels have been detected on Müller glia to participate in dispersing localized accumulation of these ions. Müller glia can also participate in regulating local parenchyma proton concentration through conversion of bicarbonate and CO_2 (Bringmann et al., 2006). They possess carbonic anhydrase II transporters. Collectively these factors influence osmotic regulation, and express aquaporin 4 (AQP4) to facilitate the diffusion of water throughout the depth of retinal tissue (Nagelhus et al., 2004).

Müller glia are being identified for their supportive role in new functions as well. This can include general trophic support, anti-oxidative glutathione production, and preventing optical dispersion passing through the retinal tissue (Reichenbach and Bringmann, 2013). They serve a very active role in maintaining retinal function and are more than a simple substrate to compose neuronal circuitry, and their function would be significantly altered with these specialized functions. In recent decades, retinal neuroscientists have had a new appreciation for their specialized function to respond to retinal damage, and potentially replace damaged or lost retinal neurons.

Species specific responses of Müller glia to retinal injury and disease

Müller glia can be identified throughout vertebrate species, and fulfill similar functions in maintaining neuronal activity and visual function. A significant difference between species is their response to retinal injury or disease. In mammals, Müller glia become reactive and gliotic, paralleling the response of astrocytes in other regions of the central nervous system. This is traditionally characterized by an upregulation of intermediate filaments, such as GFAP, nestin, and vimentin (Bringmann et al., 2009; Sofroniew, 2014). Reactive glia also secrete other cytokines, growth factors, and matrix proteins as part of this gliotic response. Reactive astrocytosis has also been characterized as A1 vs A2 profile (Liddelow et al., 2017), with these classical markers of gliosis correlating to an array of genes that fall into the aforementioned categories.

Gliotic response in Mammalian & Human Müller glia

Müller glia undergo these expression changes which can serve a beneficial role in curtailing the extent of neuronal death via neurotrophic factor secretion in damage or disease (Bringmann and Reichenbach, 2001; Hippert et al., 2015). However, these changes can also induce further tissue destruction through immune signaling cascades triggering microglia reactivity, pro-apoptotic factors, and immune cell recruitment (Sofroniew, 2005). In most cases of disease or damage, Müller glia typically do not undergo proliferation.

In humans with severe retinal damage, Müller glia play a critical role in the formation of periretinal and epiretinal membranes via pro-inflammatory factors and extracellular matrix remodeling (Sethi et al., 2005). While Müller glia typically do not proliferate under stress or disease, they do undergo proliferation after retinal detachment and in proliferative vitreoretinopathy that is believed to contribute to retinal membranes in disease(Abrams, 1997; Eastlake et al., 2016). While there is some evidence that they reduce the expression of glial genes and transition to a less differentiated state, they do not regenerate lost retinal neurons in vivo. There is some evidence that human and mammalian Müller glia can be induced into a neuronal like state in vitro (Jayaram et al., 2014; Singhal et al., 2012), but there is no evidence that post developmental neurogenesis naturally occurs.

In mice, Müller glia do not enter mitotic cycles, but can be similarly induced to proliferate under a pathological state (Dyer and Cepko, 2000). Young mice with models of proliferative vitreoretinopathy also have Müller glia proliferation and can express genes associated with retinal stem cells (Hollborn et al., 2005). This proliferative response has been correlated to an increase in epidermal growth factor (EGF) (Hollborn et al., 2005). EGF can promote postnatal mouse Müller glia to proliferate in explant cultures and to a limited degree after damage in vivo (Ueki and Reh, 2013). Similar to human Müller glia, they can be stimulated in-vivo to adopt neuronal and rod photoreceptors in-vitro (Pollak et al., 2013a).

Unlike mammalian retinas, the retinas of teleost fish have been observed to regenerate retinal neurons following injury or disease, such as goldfish, trout, flounder, and zebrafish (Cameron, 2000; Faillace et al., 2002, 200; Hitchcock, 1997; Mader and Cameron, 2004). Zebrafish became the predominant model to study this phenomenon provided their ease in maintaining colonies and genetic manipulation (Goldman, 2014). Although the retina have many similarities to mammalian counterparts, zebrafish also possess a ciliary marginal zone that contains proliferating progenitor cells that contribute to new neurons throughout the animals life, and they also contain rod precursor cells in the ONL that possess the competence to form new rod photoreceptors when stimulated for retinal repair (Goldman, 2014).

While the restorative properties of teleost fish have been observed in the mid-20th century, the origin of these damage responsive cells that serve as the precursor for regenerated neurons was unknown. Early evidence in the zebrafish existed from the tubulin 1a-GFP reporter transgenic zebrafish (Fausett and Goldman, 2006). Tubulin 1a (tuba1a) is a component gene that polymerizes to form microtubules important to cytoskeleton structure (Laferriere et al., 1997). These microtubule isoforms are most commonly expressed in differentiated neurons and neuronal progenitors, which was observed in the developing and regenerating zebrafish CNS (Senut et al., 2004). Strong evidence that Müller glia are the source of these progenitors was through lineage tracing of Müller glia that were tuba1a-GFP⁺ after focal injury (Fausett and Goldman, 2006). They used bromodeoxyuridine (BrdU), an analog of uridine that incorporates into to the new forming strand of DNA during S-phase of the cell cycle, that colocalized to traditional Müller glia markers. When tracking Brdu positive cells over several weeks, they found that all cell types had been newly formed.

Limited Avian regeneration

In response to retinal injury, the adult birds are not capable of regenerating the damaged retina. Like the zebrafish, a proliferative ciliary marginal zone was identified in the postnatal chick into adulthood (Fischer and Reh, 2000). It was observed that early in embryonic chick retinal development, that the pigmented retinal epithelium can transdifferentiate into all retinal subtypes (Coulombre and Coulombre, 1965). A pivotal finding was that in response to acute retinal damage that Müller glia began to proliferate in the central and peripheral retina as denoted by dual positive BrdU glutamine synthetase (GS) positive cells (Fischer and Reh, 2001). However, many of these cells would remain in an undifferentiated state and maintain stem factors such as Chx10 and Pax6 (Fischer and Reh, 2001). Additionally, the number of BrdU positive cells would decrease over several weeks, suggested many of these additional cells undergo attrition. Despite most cells remaining gliotic or progenitor like, a few progenitors would upregulate the expression of amacrine and bipolar markers such as HuC/D (Fischer and Reh, 2001). A subsequent study where colchicine was used to induce ganglion cell death, a few of these Müller glia derived progenitor cells (MGPC) would form into ganglion-like cells (Fischer and Reh, 2002).

This intermediate phenotype of the postnatal chick retina set the precedent for future studies using this model of regeneration. While the retina largely fails to replenish lost neurons and the majority Müller glia upregulate gliosis genes similar to that of mammalian models, there is a marginal production of progenitors that form neurons. This provides a model where cell signaling cascades can be studied using pharmacological targeting to both inhibit and potentiate the regenerative response of Müller glia. The Fischer lab has published many follow-up studies into the important signaling events that mediate the transition from mature glial cell into a progenitor cell and neurogenesis.

Signaling cascades driving Müller glia reprogramming

Provided the difference in regenerative capacity of Müller glia between species, several studies have been conducted to understand the mechanism behind the transition from glial cell to progenitor cell. With a better understanding of these regulatory cell networks, a formulated strategy to stimulating Müller glia in mammalian retina may be more successful. MAPK-signaling pathway has been repeatedly established to stimulate the formation of MGPCs in fish (Wan et al., 2012), chick (Fischer et al., 2002b), and mouse (Nakazawa et al., 2008). MAPK signaling traditionally functions through the activation of receptor tyrosine kinases which activate mitogen activated kinase kinases (MEKs) and ERK, leading to a cascade of phosphorylation including transcription factors such as Egr1 and pCREB to effectuate changes in gene expression (De Luca et al., 2012).

MAPK kinases are potent inducers of MGPC formation, and are one of the few activators of Müller glia that can sufficiently drive the transition to a progenitor cell without damage in zebrafish and chick. HB-EGF is sufficient to induce MGPCs in zebrafish without damage through MAPK signaling (Wan et al., 2012) and activation of pERK (Wan et al., 2014). Similarly in chick, FGF2 is the only known factor to induce any MGPCs in the absence of retinal damage (Fischer et al., 2002b). FGF2 and insulin treatment was observed to feed into MAPK signaling and associated effectors Egr1, cFos and pCREB (Fischer et al., 2009a; Fischer et al., 2009b). In mice, pERK and cFos are activated after damage, but no mitogenic response is observed (Nakazawa et al., 2008). The addition of FGF and EGF in combination with retinal damage can stimulate sparse formation of MGPCs in the adult mouse. This pathway has proven to be a pivotal growth factor in MG reprogramming and has conserved effects across species.

In addition to growth factors and MAPK activation, several other conserved mitogenic pathways were also observed to serve a supporting role in MGPC formation. Wnt-signaling through β-catenin is a potent mitogenic pathway that is sufficient to induce MGPCs in zebrafish without damage (Ramachandran et al., 2011), potentiate MGPC formation in damaged chick retina (Gallina et al., 2015), and potentially lead to MGPCs in undamaged mouse retina when overexpressed via adeno-associated virus (AAV) gene delivery (Yao et al., 2016). A similarly potent mitogenic pathway PI3K/Akt/mTOR-signaling was activated through signaling cross-talk in FGF2 treated chick retinas (Zelinka et al., 2016) and found to be necessary for proliferation in EGF treated mouse retinal explants (Ueki and Reh, 2013). TGFβ-Smad2/3 signaling were found to have inhibitory effects on MGPC formation in chick and zebrafish retina (Lenkowski et al., 2013; Todd et al., 2017), where Smad1/5/8 mediated BMP signaling was found to have a positive regulatory effect on the number of progenitors in the

damaged chick retina (Todd et al., 2017).

Conserved pathways important for retinal development were also found to be

important in the production of MGPCs, such as notch and sonic hedgehog. Notch

signaling is important for maintaining cell proliferation and gliogenesis in late

neurodevelopment, but was also found to be upregulated in Müller glia after damage

and necessary for MGPC production (Ghai et al., 2010). Sonic hedgehog signaling was

observed to be present in chick Müller glia, and administration of receptor agonists

increased retinal levels of Ptch1, Gli1, Gli2, Gli3, Hes1, and Hes5 and increased the

number of MGPCs after damage (Todd and Fischer, 2015).

Role of Immune Signaling in Müller glia Reprogramming

Cytokine signaling factors produced and secreted by the immune cells impact not

only other immune cells, but also glial cells (John et al., 2003). Microglia are the

resident immune cells of the retina, that are present throughout the CNS of vertebrates.

These are active cells in facilitating normal retinal development and function in addition

to classical roles of immune surveillance for injury and infection (Silverman and Wong,

2018a). They possess pathogen and damage associated molecular pattern

(PAMP/DAMP) receptors that trigger reactivity and efflux of cytokines (Kawasaki and

Kawai, 2014). In the retina, Müller glia reactivity is also sensitive to these factors and

signal through toll-like receptors (TLR) to react to tissue damage or disease (Kumar and

Shamsuddin, 2012).

Multiple studies have shown that Müller glia reprogramming is impacted by

immunomodulatory factors mediated in part my microglia. In zebrafish, photoreceptors were selectively ablated using transgenic expression of bacterial nitroreductase and administration of metronidazole, where the pro-drug is converted to a cytotoxin that kills the cell. This resulted in microglia taking on an ameboid reactive morphology and migrating to the affected photoreceptors (White et al., 2017). This was accompanied by the production of MGPCs. However, when microglia were also included in the ablation, MGPC formation was significantly impaired (White et al., 2017). This effect was reproduced using a potent anti-inflammatory glucocorticoid inhibitor before damage, dexamethasone (White et al., 2017).

Inflammatory factor TNF-α was found to also be necessary for the initial response of Müller glia to become MGPCs in the zebrafish (Nelson et al., 2013a). TNF signaling feeds into a predominant inflammatory pathways NF-kB, which is an upregulated network in zebrafish Müller glia (Sifuentes et al., 2016). Leptin, CNTF, and IL-6 family of cytokines also synergize to be able to generate MGPCs in zebrafish in the absence of damage (Nelson et al., 2012; Zhao et al., 2014a). This functions through Jak/Stat signaling (Kassen et al., 2009).

The role of microglia and cytokine signaling has found to exhibit similar patterns in the chick. When the retina is damaged, microglia become reactive and mediate IL6 signaling to influence neuronal survival (Fischer et al., 2015; Gallina et al., 2015). These cytokines are also important to MGPC production as evidenced by the ablation of microglia using clodronate liposomes results in no MGPC formation in the damaged retina (Fischer et al., 2014a). When microglia reactivity is repressed with dexamethasone, we see a similar reduction in the number of MGPCs seen in zebrafish (Gallina et al., 2014b). CNTF and damage upregulates Jak/Stat signaling which is necessary for MGPC formation (Todd et al., 2016). However, in chick these inflammatory cascades can induce opposing effects on Müller glia to form progenitor cells. Activators of NFkB signaling with retinal damage in the chick is a potent suppressor of MGPC formation (Palazzo et al., 2020b). When microglia are ablated and NFkB is activated with a TNFα homolog, MGPC formation can be restored (Palazzo et al., 2020b). Both the pathway of inflammatory activation and the timing appear to play an important role (White et al., 2017).

In mice, inflammatory signaling appears to be repressive to reprogramming and neurogenesis. In mouse models that over express stem cell factor Ascl1, Jak/Stat signaling leads to transcription factor binding to inappropriate sites that repress neurogenesis (Jorstad et al., 2020). Similarly, transcriptomic analysis suggests NFkB is a key regulator in mediating the expression of pro glial NFI transcription factors (Hoang et al., 2020). Ablating microglia in this mouse model also boosts neurogenesis from progenitor cell populations (Todd et al., 2020).

Collectively, this data suggests an important role of immune factors in coordinating a gliotic or regenerative response between species. There are an array of inflammatory cytokines and cross talk between these signaling pathways. The chapters of this book explore other potential regulators of inflammation that could both influence different cell signaling cascades, or the degree of temporal activation. This is important information to advance the field of reprogramming as a potential therapeutic strategy for retinal disease and further current mammalian models of retinal regeneration.

Limitations of current mammalian reprogramming based cell replacement

strategies

Over the past few years, several high profile publications have claimed extraordinary abilities to regenerate retinal neurons in the mouse (Blackshaw and Sanes, 2021). However, many of these studies have yet to be reproduced in other laboratories and developed further in follow-up publications. Many of these studies involve the gene delivery of constructs via AAVs. AAV capsid isoforms have the ability to infect several subtypes of neurons and Müller glia (Hickey et al., 2017; Pellissier et al., 2014). Cell specific promoters are then utilized to induce the expression of the transgene in the cell type of interest. This has been used on Müller glia to induce neuronal differentiation of 1) rod photoreceptors with Otx, Crx, and Nrl overexpression (Yao et al., 2018), ganglion cells with Ptbp1 knockdown (Zhou et al., 2020), or ganglion cells from Math5, Brn3 overexpression (Xiao et al., 2019). Many of these studies also include light responsiveness and functional recovery with their regenerated cells (Yao et al., 2018; Zhou et al., 2020). With these supposed advancements in the generation of retinal neurons, the necessity to explore other regulators or supporting factors in reprogramming rather than advance the most effective technique would be in question.

After the publication of these findings, criticism has been raised of these high impact papers from other senior researchers in the field (Blackshaw and Sanes, 2021). While faults in scientific rigor may account for differential findings, such as ptbp1 inducing ganglion cells (Zhou et al., 2020) in one lab and photoreceptors in another (Fu et al., 2020), overstated conclusions may be due to faulty interpretations from the implemented methodology (Wang et al., 2020). While minipromoters delivered by adeno-associated viruses (AAVs) may convey cell specificity in the short term, a GFAP mini-promoter was activated in neurons after several weeks (Wang et al., 2020). The serotype of the virus determined the population of infected cells where the majority were astrocytes, some infected cells were neurons. Hence, the minipromoter was unexpectedly activated ectopically in neurons. Furthermore, the tropism of the virus was likely also influenced by the side of the DNA insert delivered, as longer plasmids with NeuroD1 activated different populations of endogenous cells after several weeks (Wang et al., 2020).

This approach is still in its infancy as a potential translatable therapeutic, and some new developments that have elicited excitement in current years may be overstated. Some models have withstood scrutiny, such as the ASCL1 over expressing mice, that are capable of producing circuit integrating interneurons when stimulated with damage and histone deacetylase inhibitor trichostatin A (Jorstad et al., 2017; Pollak et al., 2013a, 1). Unlike the aforementioned studies, this is a transgenic mouse line with established cell-specific promotors that are activated by Cre recombinase and has been validated with unbiased single cell RNA sequencing (scRNA-seq) screenings (Jorstad et al., 2020; Todd et al., 2020). scRNA-seq provides the ability to screen the transcriptomic changes that occur during either transdifferentiation or reprogramming through a progenitor-like state. Phenomenology that occurs due to methodology will be corrective with this rapidly developing tool that has become prevalent in studies in cellular biology. Chapters in this book utilize this tool to both unbiasly screen new candidates for reprogramming and reinforce the causative impact a treatment has on reprogramming.

Evolving single cell methodology in Müller glia research

Single cell sequencing came to prominence in the past 10 years as an advancement over bulk tissue sequencing where there was the ability to distinguish heterogeneity among individual cells. The adoption of the technique was limited by the cost of library construction and sequencing. Advancements of next-generation parallel sequencing techniques have vastly improved the speed, quantity, and cost of large-scale sequencing. The first mammalian single cell transcriptome was performed in 2009 (Tang et al., 2009). Given the limited number of cells capable of being captured and sequencing, many biomedical applications evolved elaborate techniques to capture abundant and rare cell types, such as serial dilution, flow sorting, robotic micromanipulation, and laser-capture.(Wang and Navin, 2015). In 2014, they developed the technique of adding a unique molecular identifier (UMI) during library amplification to allow the process to become quantitative (Islam et al., 2014). With large datasets, there has also been a concurrent evolution in the methodology to analyze the bioinformatic data and extract patterns between cells and genes.

10x Genomics 3' Single Cell Sequencing Pipeline

The 10x Genomics single cell sequencing platform is the most popular pipeline for conducting single cell sequencing analysis. The primary advantages of the method are the extensive documentation, simplified reagent kits and protocol, and the expansive developments in the bioinformatic tools to improve their accessibility to more labs. For quantitative analysis of mRNA transcripts, the 3' amplified approach is preferred. The limitations of this preparation are that 1) only transcripts that are polyadenylated will be captured (thus excluding lcRNAs and miRNAs), and that the library will only represent the 3' end of the transcript, preventing effective analysis of mRNA splicing variations.

Cells from the desired tissue must be dissociated into a single cell suspension and loaded into the 10x Chromium Controller, which is a microfluidic chip that mixes the cells, reverse transcriptase reagents with DNA primer conjugated gel beads, and emulsion oil. This creates droplets in emulsion that contain both a single cell and a single gel bead. When placed into a thermocycler, this allows parallel cDNA amplification of single cells. The gel beads contain a polydT sequence ligates to polyA tails to initiate reverse transcription. 5' to the polydT is a 16-nucleotide sequence that is unique to that gel bead that serves as a cell specific bar code. Each primer also contains a 12 nucleotide 5' UMI, that creates a unique barcode for each mRNA transcript.

The library is fragmented and indexed for Illumina next generation sequencing platforms. The Illumina produces a binary base call (BCL) file, which can then be converted into a FASTQ format, which contains sequence run metadata, the DNA sequence, and quality scores for each nucleotide. 10x Genomics developed freeware called CellRanger, which will intake FASTQ files, and parse the data into a matrix of cell IDs and gene transcripts derived from your preferred reference genome. To find patterns and visualize the data, software packages have been developed in R, such as Seurat (Satija et al., 2015) and Monocle (Trapnell et al., 2012), python's SCANPY (Wolf et al., 2018), or a standalone software developed by 10x called Loupe Browser. The most popular methodology for visualization of similarities in gene expression between cells is t-distributed stochastic neighbor embedding (tSNE) and uniform manifold approximation and projection (UMAP), where cells are placed in two-dimensional space based on pattern similarities in gene expression (McInnes et al., 2018). UMAP has become the most popular method due to its ability to scale to larger datasets and improved accuracy of global architecture of all the embedded cells. Modeling the transition of asynchronous cells is called a pseudotime projection, made possible by the improved UMAP embedding (Trapnell et al., 2014). Cells can be further characterized into clusters and gene expression visualized using heat maps and violin plots.

Single cell sequencing has become the gold standard in retinal regeneration biology. Labs have archived detailed scRNA-seq libraries of the developing retina, and comprehensive characterization of neuronal subtype variation in the mouse retina (Clark et al., 2019). This has also been performed on the epigenetic landscape of the developing retina as well (Aldiri et al., 2017; Norrie et al., 2019). Comprehensive catalogs of reprogramming in zebrafish, chick, and zebrafish during stages of reprogramming have given insight into species differences in Müller glia (Hoang et al., 2020). More libraries have also been constructed in the developmental chick retina to further characterize the distinct phenotype of retinal neurons (Yamagata et al., 2021). New data impacting MPGC formation can also be validated using scRNA-seq and query secondary targets of reprogramming (Campbell et al., 2019; Campbell et al.; Palazzo et al., 2020b). The data detailed in the upcoming chapters utilize this methodology to gain further insight into the relationship between novel effectors of MGPCs and their effect on microglia and immune signaling.

Chapter 2

Matrix-metalloproteinase expression and gelatinase activity in the avian retina and their influence on Müller glia proliferation

Introduction

The retinal extracellular matrix (ECM) consists of glycoproteins and proteoglycans that are primary components of local cellular microenvironment within the retina. The ECM composition can have a significant impact on intercellular signaling. Signaling pathways that are important for proliferation, migration, and differentiation such as Wnt/β-catenin, sonic hedgehog, and fibroblast growth factors (FGFs) are influenced by ECM mutations of heparan sulfate in *Drosophila* development (Lin, 2004). The importance of the ECM in retinal function is implicated by collagen mutations manifesting as retinal malformation and dysfunction such as Knobloch's syndrome (collagen XVIII), Alport syndrome (collagen IV), and Kniest dysplasia (collagen II) (Ihanamäki et al., 2004). The ECM is dynamically modified and replaced through tightly regulated extracellular enzymes known as matrix metalloproteinases (MMPs).

MMPs are a family of zinc^{2+} dependent proteases responsible for the degradation of the extracellular matrix. MMPs can be subdivided into categories by preferred substrates and structures including collagenases, gelatinases, stromelysins, and MT
(membrane tethered)-MMPs, and others (Iyer et al., 2012; Nagase et al., 2006). Regulation of MMP enzymatic activity is required for appropriate physiologic function. The kinetics of enzymatic activity of MMPs are regulated by phosphorylation, proteolysis, and expression of endogenous glycoprotein tissue inhibitor of matrix metalloproteinases (TIMPs) (Chakraborti et al., 2003; Nagase and Woessner, 1999). MMP2 and MMP-9 are secreted as pro-enzymes with fibronectin like repeats and a

zinc-dependent catalytic domains that have substrate specificity for gelatin, fibronectin, and collagen IV & V (Nagase et al., 2006). MMPs have been studied during ocular development in frog (*Xenopus laevis*), zebrafish (*Danio rerio*), and chicken (*Gallus domesticus*) animal models (Fitch et al., 2005; Hehr et al., 2005; Zhang et al., 2003). Abnormal MMP function has been implicated in retinal disease. For example, Sorby's macular dystrophy, an autosomal dominant form of early macular degeneration in humans, can result from a mutation in TIMP3 (Christensen et al., 2017; Qi et al., 2002). Gelatinase activity has also been implicated in other ocular pathology such as diabetic retinopathy, glaucoma, corneal neovascularization, and uveal melanoma metastasis (Logan et al., 2007; Mohammad and Kowluru, 2010; Sahay et al., 2017; Väisänen et al., 1999).

There may be important roles for gelatinases in neurogenesis and glial reprogramming in the formation of Müller glia-derived progenitor cells (MGPCs). Müller Glia (MG) serve as the primary macroglia of the retina providing neuronal support including potassium siphoning, neurotransmitter recycling, bicarbonate regulation, osmotic balance, structural support, and more (Bringmann et al., 2006; Reichenbach and Bringmann, 2013). Importantly, MG are capable of reprogramming into retinal progenitor cells and undergo neurogenesis to replace damaged neurons (Goldman, 2014). The capacity for neurogenesis, however, is species-specific. Damage to mouse retina fails to elicit significant glial reprogramming and neuronal regeneration, whereas damage to zebrafish retina results in wide-spread reprogramming of MG into progenitors that are capable of regenerating functional retinal tissue (Karl and Reh, 2010; Wan and Goldman, 2016). Chick MG have an intermediate capacity for reprogramming where MG form proliferating MGPCs with limited neurogenesis, serving as an ideal model for determining inhibiting and potentiating factors of retinal regeneration (Fischer, 2005; Fischer and Reh, 2001; Gallina et al., 2014a).

MMPs have been implicated in the reprogramming of MG. For example, epidermal growth factor (EGF) is secreted as a propeptide that requires MMP proteolytic activation, and the proliferative effect of EGF is inhibited by pan-MMP inhibitor GM6001 and restored with active EGF (Wan et al., 2012). Similarly, MMP-9 has increased expression in zebrafish retina 24 hours after injury and increases expression of ASCL1a (Achaete-Scute Homologue-1), a transcription factor that is required for the formation of MGPCs (Kaur et al., 2018). In *Xenopus* regeneration models, inhibition of MMPs suppresses the proliferation of the RPE in the formation of neuroepithelial tissue (Naitoh et al., 2017). In the avian retina, the expression and function of gelatinases are poorly characterized and have not been studied in the context of retinal regeneration.

In this study, we characterize TIMP and MMP expression and gelatinase activity in the chick retina. Furthermore, we investigate changes in gelatinase expression and activity in response to excitotoxic retinal damage. Collectively, our findings indicate that glia produce MMP2, TIMP2, and TIMP3. Interestingly, gelatinase activity decreased after retinal damage. MG were found to increase the expression of TIMP2 after damage that was localized to rod bipolar cells. Intraocular injections of gelatinase inhibitors increased the formation of proliferating MGPCs in damaged and FGF2-treated retinas.

Materials and methods

Animals:

Animals used in this study were managed in accordance with the guidelines provided by the NIH and IACUC at the Ohio State University. All chickens (*Gallus gallus domesticus*; white leghorn strain) were obtained at P0 from Meyer Hatchery (Polk, Ohio). The chicks were housed in a stainless-steel brooder maintained at 25°C with a 12-hour light and dark cycle (8am-8pm). Chicks were fed water and Purina chick starter *ad libitum*.

Preparation of clodronate liposomes:

The production of clodronate liposomes was modified from previous descriptions (Van Rooijen, 1989; Zelinka et al., 2012). Briefly, 8 mg of L-α-Phosphatidyl-DL-glycerol sodium salt (Sigma P8318) was dissolved in chloroform. 50 mg of cholesterol dissolved in chloroform was added to the lipids and evaporated under nitrogen/vacuum with frequent shaking to create a thin lipid-film on a round bottom flask. 158 mg dichloro-methylene diphosphonate (clodronate; Sigma-Aldrich) in sterile PBS was added and mixed. To facilitate lipid rehydration, the vial was vortexed for 5 minutes. To normalize lipid vesicle size, the mixture was sonicated at 42,000 Hz for 6 minutes. The liposomes were centrifuged at 10,000 x g for 15 minutes, aspirated, and resuspended in 150 μl PBS. While there is some loss of liposomes during the purification, the dosage has been tittered such that >99% of the microglia are ablated 2 days after administration.

Intraocular injections:

Intraocular injections of anesthetized chickens were conducted as previously

described (Fischer et al., 1998; Fischer et al., 2009a). Briefly, prior to injection chicks

were anesthetized via inhalation of 2.5% isoflurane and oxygen. The right eye was

treated with experimental compound and the contralateral left eye received vehicle

control in each paradigm. Each injection was 20 µl with the addition of 0.05 mg/ml

bovine serum albumen as a carrier for dilute recombinant protein injections. Information

and concentrations of all compounds injected into the eyes of the chicks is provided in

Table 2.

ScRNA-seq

Chick retinas were dissected, the pigmented epithelium was carefully removed,

and dissociation performed in a 0.25% papain solution of Hank's balanced salt solution,

pH = 7.4, for 30 minutes with frequent trituration. Dissociated cells were assessed for

viability and density and diluted to 700 cell/µl with the goal establishing a single cell

cDNA library of 10,000 cells per preparation. Cells and Chromium Single Cell 3' V2

reagents (10X Genomics) were loaded onto chips for nanodroplet packaging in the 10x

Chromium Controller. In accordance with 10x Genomics instructions, cDNA and library

amplification was achieved by 12 and 10 cycles respectively. Sequencing was

conducted on Illumina HiSeq2500 (Genomics Resource Core Facility, John's Hopkins

University) with 26 bp for Read 1 and 98 bp for Read 2. Fasta sequencing files were

aligned, de-multiplexed, annotated to the ENSMBLE database, counted for expression

levels, and gene-cell matrices were constructed. Using Cell Browser software (10x

Genomics), t-distributed stochastic neighbor embedding (tSNE) plots were generated from aggregates of multiple scRNA-seq libraries. Compiled in each tSNE plot are two biological replicates for saline injected retinas, 24 hrs, 48 hrs, and 72 hrs after NMDA damage. Identification of different types of retinal cells that were clustered together in tSNE plots was accomplished by probing for well-established cell-distinguishing genes. Seurat was used to construct violin/scatter plots (Butler et al., 2018) and Monocle was used to construct pseudo-time trajectories and scatter plotters for Müller glia and MGPCs (Qiu et al., 2017a; Qiu et al., 2017b; Trapnell et al., 2014).

Fixation, sectioning, and immunocytochemistry

Retinal samples were fixed, sectioned, and immunolabeled as previously described (Fischer et al., 2008; Gallina et al., 2014a; Gallina et al., 2015). All primary antibodies used in this study are described in Table 2.1. The following secondary antibodies are included in this study: donkey-anti-goat-Alexa488/568, goat-anti-rabbit-Alexa488/568 and goat-anti-mouse-Alexa488/568/647 (Thermo Fisher Scientific). Secondary antibodies are diluted in pH 7.4 PBS plus 0.2% Triton-X and washed in pH 7.4 PBS. Secondaries did not produce non-specific labeling in the retina and tissue sections were devoid of autofluorescence.

Tissue encapsulation and measurement of MMP activity

Each retina was cut into three replicates of 2 mm x 2 mm and weighed using an analytical balance. A hydrogel precursor solution was prepared as described previously with slight modification (Leight et al., 2013). Briefly, eight-arm 40-kDa poly (ethylene) glycol hydroxyl (JenKem Technologies) was functionalized with 5-norbornene-2-

carboxylic acid (Sigma) to form poly (ethylene) glycol-norbornene (PEG-NB) (Fairbanks et al., 2009). The PEG-NB (20 mM) macromer was crosslinked with a bicysteine MMP-degradable peptide (KCGPQG↓IWGQCK, 10.75 mM peptide; GenScript) in the presence of the photoinitiator, lithium phenyl-2, 4, 6-trimethylbenzoylphosphinate (LAP, 2 mM). CRGDS (GenScript), a cell adhesion peptide, was also included at a concentration of 1 mM. MMP activity was measured by incorporation of an MMP-degradable peptide (GGPQG↓IWGQK$_{Dde}$(PEG)$_2$C, 0.25 mM) conjugated with a fluorophore (Fluorescein; Life Technologies) and quencher (Dabcyl; AnaSpec) pair. Ten microliters of the hydrogel precursor solution were pipetted into a 96-well, round-bottom, black plate (BrandTech). Tissue samples were immersed into the hydrogel solution and polymerized under 4 mW/cm^2 UV light (365 nm) for 3 min. 150 µL of DMEM:F12 media (Life Technologies) supplemented with 1% (v/v) charcoal-stripped FBS (VWR), 1% penicillin/streptomycin and 1% L-glutamine were added to each well. Plates were incubated at 37 °C, 5% CO$_2$. 18 hours post-encapsulation, AlamarBlue (LifeTechnologies) reagent (1:10) was added to each well to measure tissue metabolic activity. Fluorescence measurements of the MMP-degradable peptide (494 nm excitation/521 nm emission) and AlamarBlue (560 nm excitation/590 nm emission) were made simultaneously in each well at 24 hours after encapsulation with a 3 x 3 well scan using a Molecular Devices SpectraMax M2 spectrophotometer. Readings of average fluorescence intensity were calculated for each well scan and the background reading (peptide-functionalized gels containing no tissue samples) was subtracted. All fluorescence intensity measurements were normalized to sample mass or metabolic activity and averaged between replicates.

In situ zymography staining

Retinal tissue was fixed for 48hrs at room temperature (RT) in zinc-based fixative consisting of 36.7mM $ZnCl_2$ (Sigma-Aldrich, St. Louis, MO), 27.3mM $ZnAc_2$ x $2H_2O$ (MP Biomedicals, Santa Ana, CA), and 0.63mM $CaAc_2$ (Spectrum Chemical MFG Corp, New Brunswick, NJ) dissolved in 0.1M Tris-HCl (Sigma-Aldrich), pH 7.4. OCT embedded retinas were sectioned (20 µm), air dried at RT for at least one hour, and rinsed with deionized water to remove excess OCT. Sections were then incubated in a humidity chamber at 37°C for 1hr with either 200µM 1,10-Phenanthroline (Sigma-Aldrich) diluted in water (MMP inhibitor control), or at 4°C for 1hr (temperature control). After incubation, solutions were removed and 20µg/mL fluorescein conjugated dye quenched (DQ) gelatin from pig skin (Life Technologies, Carlsbad, CA), ±200µM 1,10-Phenanthroline, was diluted in reaction buffer [10mM Tris-HCl, 30mM NaCl (Fisher Scientific, Waltham, MA), 1mM $CaCl_2$ (Fisher Scientific), and 0.04mM sodium azide (Fisher Scientific). Sections were then incubated at 37°C or 4°C for 2hr in a dark humidity chamber. Slides were rinsed in water then fixed with 4% neutral buffered formalin for 10min at RT and then rinsed with phosphate buffered saline (PBS, Gibco, Waltham, MA) twice, for 2min each. Nuclei were then stained with 1:1000 Hoechst 33342 (Life Technologies) in PBS for 30min at RT. Slides were mounted using ProLong Gold antifade reagent (Invitrogen, Carlsbad, CA).

Photography, measurements, cell counts and statistics:

Microscopy images were captured with the Leica DM5000B microscope with epifluorescence and the Leica DC500 digital camera. Confocal images were obtained with a Leica SP8 in The Department of Neuroscience Imaging Facility at The Ohio State University. Representative images have enhanced color, brightness, and contrast for improved clarity using Adobe Photoshop. In proliferation assays, a fixed area of retina was captured and quantified for Sox2 and Edu colocalization. The region of the retina was selected and standardized between treatment and control groups to reduce variability and improve reproducibility.

For quantifying changes in context specific protein expression, densitometry measurements of fluorescent immunohistological stains were compared. Within each image, the retina was stratified into the photoreceptor layer (PRL), outer (photoreceptor) nuclear layer (ONL), outer plexiform layer (OPL), inner nuclear layer (INL), inner plexiform layer (IPL), ganglion cell layer (GCL), and the nerve fiber layer (NFL). Within each layer, a region of retina was selected and mean pixel intensity (0-255) was derived. This process was repeated 3 times within each selected image, and the whole process was repeated for each biological replicate. ImagePro 6.2, ImageJ, and Microsoft Excel were used for data and calculations respectively.

To calculate changes in spatial distribution, the image was subjected to a consistent threshold value to remove background. The average area of distribution beginning at the IPL bordering the INL was derived and plotted for each pixel throughout the layer for each retina. The relative distance of each pixel was derived from the confocal scalebar corresponding to the magnification and image resolution. All data was calculated using ImageJ.

For statistical evaluation of differences in treatments, a two-tailed paired T-test was applied for intra-individual variability where each biological sample also served as its own control. For two treatment groups comparing inter-individual variability, a standard two-tailed unpaired T-test was applied. For multivariate analysis, an ANOVA with the associated Tukey Test was used to evaluate any significant differences between multiple groups.

Results

Gelatinase activity decreases in the NMDA damaged chick retina

MMPs have been characterized in both physiologic and pathologic models of retinal disease. MMPs are translated as pro-peptides subject to complex and dynamic regulation including trafficking, proteolytic activation, enzymatic inhibition, and degradation. We directly measured gelatinase activity in tissue sections of the retina using *in situ* zymography (Fig. 2.1). MMP activity was localized to specific layers of the retina using *in situ* zymography where DQ-gelatin was cleaved (Fig. 2.1A). For example, within the inner INL there was elevated gelatinase activity corresponding to the location of cell bodies of Müller glia and amacrine cells (Fig. 2.1B). Across multiple biological replicates, gelatinase activity was stratified into three relative levels of activity – high, medium, and low (Fig. 2.1C) – that were significantly different from each other ($p < 0.05$). The highest gelatinase activity was found in the ONL, IPL, and NFL, followed by the PRL, INL, and GCL. The lowest level of MMP activity was found in the IPL.

We investigated how gelatinase activity may change in the retina following NMDA-induced damage. Retinal tissue was incubated in a fluorescein conjugated DQ-peptide hydrogel that measured changes in gelatinase enzymatic activity through spectrophotometry. Retinal tissue gelatinase activity was unchanged 4 hours after damage *in vitro*, but steadily decreased over the following 48 hours relative to that seen

in saline-treated controls (Fig. 2.1D, E). Gelatinase activity began to increase after 48

hours but remained reduced at 7 days after damage when measured against saline

injected retinas (Fig. 2.2D,E). This trend was consistent when data was standardized to

total tissue metabolic activity or collagenase enzyme activity (total matrix degradation,

positive control).

In situ techniques were performed to determine layer-specific changes in

gelatinase activity. Densitometry measurements of gelatinase activity across all layers

of the retina were not sensitive enough to detect significant changes after NMDA

damage (data not shown). To investigate further, measurements of gelatinase activity

were performed for each retinal layer after NMDA damage. In the IPL at the 4 and 24

hours after damage, gelatinase activity was decreased, but later increased at 72 hours

after damage (Fig. 2.2F). Conversely, gelatinase activity in the GCL was slightly

elevated 24, 48, and 72 hours after damage (Fig. 2.2F). At the 7-day time point,

gelatinase activity across all layers was not significantly different to that of the control

undamaged retinas (Fig. 2.2F).

Single-cell RNA-seq: MMPs and TIMPs in normal and damaged retinas

To identify the different cell types that express gelatinases and other MMPs in

the avian retina, we created scRNA-seq libraries of control and NMDA-damaged retinas

(Fig. 2.2). Each library of undamaged and NMDA damaged retinas consisted of two

biological replicates. For tSNE plot analysis, an aggregate library was generated

consisting of control undamaged retinas and retinas collected 24, 48, and 72 hours following NMDA damage. Using well-established cell markers, tSNE-clustered cells were identified as different types of retinal cells (Fig. 2.2A,B). Different types of MMPs were detected in the different types of cells in the chick retina. Of note, MMP2 was identified in NIRG cells and oligodendrocytes, whereas MMP-9 was only detected at low levels in amacrine, NIRG cells, and Müller glia (Fig. 2.2C,D). Although reports have previously claimed that microglia are a source of gelatinases in the CNS in response to ischemia and inflammation (Könnecke and Bechmann, 2013), our scRNA-seq library indicates that microglia are not the primary source of MMP2 in the retina.

Other MMPs detected in the chick retina included membrane bound MMPs 15, 16, and 24 (MT2, MT3, MT5-MMP) in Müller glia and different neuronal cell types at lower levels (Fig. 2.2E-I). The expression of MMP16 and MMP24 was seen at detection threshold for the 10X V2 reagents and was only observed in a small proportion of MG in control, 24hr, 48hr, and 72hrs after damage. The proportion of MG positive for MMP16 and MMP24 did not change after damage (4.24% and 2.78% of MG for MMP16 and MMP24 respectively). While MMP24 was always observed at low levels, the proportion of positive cells was noticeably increased in amacrine and ganglion cells (6.16% and 17.17% respectively). Pseudotime analysis indicated that the relative levels of MMP16 and MMP24 expression were higher in resting and activated Müller glia, but decreased along the pseudotime trajectory toward MGPCs (Fig. 2.2J). Lastly, MMPs 7, 11, 13, and 28 showed no expression in any cell type.

Inhibition of gelatinases enhances MGPC proliferation.

Since we observed transient decreases in gelatinase activity following NMDA

damage, where MGPCs are known to form, we investigated whether gelatinase

inhibitors affected the reprogramming of Müller glia in to proliferating MGPCs.

Administration of gelatinase inhibitor SB-3CT at the time of damage did not influence

the formation of MGPCs (data not shown). By comparison, administration of SB-3CT

prior to damage significantly increased numbers of proliferating MGPCs (Fig. 2.3A,B).

This proliferative effect was only seen in Müller glia, and not NIRG cells or microglia

(Fig. 2.3C,D). Similarly, the MMP2-specific inhibitor MMP2i II applied before NMDA

resulted in significant increases in numbers of proliferating MGPCs, whereas the

proliferation of NIRG cells and microglia was unaffected (Fig. 2.3E,F,H,I). By contrast,

the MMP-9 specific MMP-9i-I inhibitor had no significant effect upon the proliferation of

cells in damaged retinas (Fig. 2.3G).

In the retina, damage can induce dramatic changes in extracellular matrix which

may lead to an effect of NMDA only in the context of retinal cell death. With both SB-

3CT and MMP2i-II, cell death was measured by terminal deoxynucleotidyl transferase

dUTP nick end labeling (TUNEL) and ratio of ONL/INL thickness (Fig. 2.10). There was

no influence on amacrine cell death compared to control.

Provided that reducing gelatinase activity increased proliferation in response to

NMDA damage, we sought to investigate how reducing gelatinase activity influences the

formation of proliferating MGPCs in retinas treated with FGF2 in the absence of

damage. The combination of insulin and FGF2 is known to induce a wave of MGPC

formation, initiating at the far periphery of the retina (Fischer and Bongini, 2010; Fischer

et al., 2002b). Using a similar injection paradigm, both SB-3CT and MMP2i II inhibitors resulted in significant increases in numbers of proliferating MGPCs in FGF2-treated retinas (Fig. 2.4A,B,C). The proliferation of NIRG cells and microglia was not affected by the MMP inhibitors (Fig. 2.4D,E). In conjunction with the observation of increased proliferation, FGF2 treated retinas showed an increase response of cFos expression in Müller glia after the treatment of SB-3CT (Fig. 2.4F,G).

TIMP expression in damaged retinas and the formation of MGPCs:

Observing the high expression of TIMP2 and TIMP3 mRNA in the retina, we investigated changes in mRNA expression following damage in both Müller glia and NIRG populations (Fig. 2.5). The scRNA-seq retinal library revealed distinct cell types from clustering in a tSNE plot (Fig. 2.5A). Müller glia to MGPCs were identified based on elevated expression of Ascl1, Nestin, Rax1, PCNA, and Cdk1 (Fig. 2.5,B). The aggregate tSNE plot included two biological replicates of undamaged, 24, 48, and 72 hours following NMDA damage. TIMP2 expression in each cell is displayed as a heat map with deep red indicating high expression on a $\log_2$ scale from 0 to 4.1 (Fig. 2.5C). Müller glia with expression levels above 4-fold are labeled white, showing an increased population of high expression TIMP2 in Müller glia 24 hrs after damage and in forming MGPCs (Fig. 2.5D,E,F,G). Similarly, TIMP3 expression increased in NIRG cells after damage, with the greatest population of NIRGS expressing TIMP3 24 hours after NMDA damage (Fig. 2.5H,I).

TIMP2 localizes to inner retinal neurons and is altered after NMDA damage.

TIMP2 mRNA was high in Müller glia and the expression was increased after NMDA damage. Since TIMPs are secreted from cells, we used antibodies to investigate where these proteins might act (Cawston et al., 1983; Howard et al., 1991; Welgus et al., 1985). TIMP2 is a secreted protein and has been associated with cell surface proteins with local MMP inhibition (Butler et al., 1998; Emmert-Buck et al., 1995, 2; Itoh et al., 1998). In undamaged chick retina, TIMP2-immunolabeling is localized to every layer of the retina except the PRL, GCL, and the NFL (Fig. 2.6A). While TIMP2 mRNA was detected predominantly in Müller glia, TIMP2 protein was localized predominantly to neuronal cells (Fig. 2.6A). Low levels of TIMP2-immunoreactivity were colocalized in regions of GS-positive Muller glia, most notably in the sclerad half of the INL and MG end feet projections into the ONL (Fig. 2.6B,C). With this exception, TIMP2 demonstrated the highest intensity on neuronal cells, and did not display MG process morphology or GS colocalization in the IPL.

Because bipolar cell projections travel in fasciculi through the INL, it is challenging to delineate bipolar cell subsets that colocalize with TIMP2. Bipolar cells that accumulated serotonin did not display TIMP2-immunoreactivity on projections in the INL or IPL (Fig. 2.6D,E). While there was TIMP2 overlap within a fasciculus, tracking individual neurite projections did not colocalize with TIMP2 (Fig. 2.6F,G,H,I). Into the IPL there was little to no overlap and serotonergic bipolar cells which terminated on a different ON layer than the TIMP2 positive bipolar cells. PKCα, a rod specific bipolar cell marker, was found to co-label for TIMP2 in both the INL and the IPL (Fig. 2.6F,G,H,I). These patterns were quantifiably consistent among many bipolar cell projections across the retina (Fig. 2.11).

TIMP2 protein is cleared from the IPL early after NMDA damage

The pattern of TIMP2 localization was significantly altered in the IPL from 4 to 48 hours after NMDA damage (Fig. 2.7). 24 hours after damage, TIMP2 was at its minimal level and returned to control levels 72 hours after damage (Fig. 2.7A,B). To further analyze TIMP2 in the IPL, we characterized immunolabeling above threshold to identify TIMP2$^+$ neurites (Fig. 2.7C,D). The TIMP2-immunoreactivity was greatest near the borders of the INL and the GCL in undamaged retinas (Fig. 2.7E). In damaged retinas, early changes included the expansion of IPL and the loss of the proximal GCL border TIMP2$^+$ neurites. Edemic swelling of the of IPL following treatment of the retina with excitotoxins has been well characterized (Fischer et al., 1998). By 24 hours, TIMP2-immunoreactivity was limited to the INL/IPL border. TIMP2-immunoreactivity re-appeared in the IPL by 48 hours after damage but did not regain the distribution seen in control retinas by 72 hours.

The decrease in IPL TIMP2 correlates with the decrease in IPL gelatinase activity (Fig. 2.2F), leading to the hypothesis that TIMP2 may be an enzymatic activator of MMP-2. Therefore, we predicted that exogenous addition of TIMP2 may dampen the regenerative response of MG following NMDA damage. Indeed, intravitreal TIMP2 statistically reduced the formation of MGPCs 3 days after NMDA damage, measured by the decrease in Sox2$^+$ Edu$^+$ per retinal field (Fig. 2.7 F,G).

Microglia influence retinal TIMP2 and TIMP3 after NMDA damage

Microglia can influence the neuroinflammatory microenvironment of the retina and these glial cells are activated in response to NMDA damage. To determine whether microglia regulate gelatinase activity in retinal tissue, we compared retinal responses to NMDA damage after microglial ablation. The ablation of microglia was accomplished by delivery of clodronate liposomes, which results in >99% microglial death (Fischer et al., 2014b). Single cell sequencing indicated an increase in TIMP3 with NIRG cells maximally at 24hrs after damage, and when this experiment is repeated without retinal microglia, the production of TIMP3 is dampened (Fig. 2.8A). However, TIMP2 protein distribution or mRNA production by MG were not affected by the absence of microglia 24 hrs after damage (Fig. 2.8C, D).

The *in vitro* gelatinase enzymatic activity was also compared to NMDA-damaged retinas with or without microglia. When comparing the change in gelatinase activity, NMDA induced a reproducible decrease in gelatinase activity when microglia were present (Fig. 2.8E, F). When microglia were ablated, NMDA did not induce a significant decrease the gelatinase activity (Fig. 2.8E, F). When standardizing the activity to the mass of the retinal tissue, there was a significant decrease in gelatinase activity observed with microglial ablation alone (Fig. 2.8F). When normalized to metabolic activity, the reduction in reactive microglia are presumed to cause an average decrease in metabolic activity, potentially overestimating the standardized value and masking the pro-gelatinase role of microglia in the undamaged retina.

Discussion

This study focused on characterizing gelatinase activity in retinal tissue *in vitro* and *in situ*, and the ability to modulate enzymatic activity to influence MGPC formation. Specifically, MMP2 was produced by oligodendrocytes and NIRG cells, a secretive process potentially regulated by microglia in the retina. Gelatinase activity decreased in the natural response to NMDA damage, and when MMP2 was inhibited through two different small molecule drugs, MGPC formation can be potentiated. In trying to understand the factors modulating gelatinase activity and its influence on MG reprogramming, we suggest that TIMP2 and TIMP3 dynamics are changing in response to NMDA damage to influence the reprogramming microenvironment and potentiate MGPC formation.

Retinal gelatinases and enzymatic activity

Gelatinase activity was characterized in the avian retina by detecting and quantifying active enzymatic activity. Due to the multivariate levels of regulation involved in balancing the enzyme kinetics *in vivo*, an analysis of MMP2 and MMP-9 enzymatic activity is the best measure to determine their role in physiologic homeostatic function. Cleavage of a fluorescein quenching peptide polymerized into a tissue stabilizing hydrogel can be used quantitatively to infer both temporal and spatial changes in MMP activity (Leight et al., 2013; Shin et al., 2018).

We report that retinal tissue expresses predominantly MMP2, not MMP-9, and that the origins of synthesis are in oligodendrocytes and NIRG cells. In the CNS, a commonly believed source of gelatinases are microglia, which have been demonstrated to secrete MMPs in other animals in the context of neuroinflammation and injury (Nuttall et al., 2007; Rosenberg, 2002; Yamada et al., 1995). Our scRNA-seq analysis of microglia does not show gelatinase transcription with or without damage. While the absence of detectable transcripts may be a biproduct of limited microglia extraction, or below detection thresholds as a low copy transcript, our data suggests that microglia play a role in maintaining gelatinase levels as enzyme activity decreases after damage. Hence, retinal microglia may play an indirect role through paracrine signaling to other glia or secreting other non-gelatinase factors.

Each layer in the retina was found to have a varying degree of gelatinase activity, and the stratified pattern suggests complex gelatinase regulation. Interestingly, the INL had an intermediate gelatinase activity that was detected on a gradient, with lower gelatinase activity in the outer INL (sclerad surface) and a higher level in the inner INL (vitread surface). The highest activity was seen paracellularly surrounding DAPI nuclei, suggesting that cell surface proteases modulate their localized activity. MMP2 can be bound and localized to the cell surface by integrin $\alpha v\beta 3$ (found on MG, data not shown), and further activated by membrane type (MT) MMPs (Brooks et al., 1996; Emmert-Buck et al., 1995; Llano et al., 1999; Zhao et al., 2004). For example, our scRNA-seq data indicate MMP24 expression in amacrine cells, which may explain why the vitread half of the INL has more gelatinase activity than the sclerad half of the INL. After damage, pseudotime plots indicate there was a declining trend of cell surface MMPs 16 and 24 as MG made the transition into progenitor cells. While this did not appear to affect the total INL gelatinase activity, this may affect the ECM microenvironment of MGPCs and subsequent autocrine and paracrine signaling.

The pattern of gelatinase activity likely represents an aggregate of multiple sources of gelatinases found in proximity of the tissue such as the retinal pigmented epithelium (RPE). In chick MMP2 expression has previously been detected in the RPE and in the photoreceptor layer (Takeyama et al., 2010). Although our scRNA-seq data do not support the notion that photoreceptors contribute gelatinases, secretion by the RPE, or perhaps Müller glia, would explain the origins of high enzymatic activity within the PRL, OPL, and ONL. Gelatinases near the vitread surface of the retina may originate from resident macrophages and monocytes present in the vitreous chamber of the eye. These cell types have been demonstrated to express gelatinases, with supporting evidence of MMP secretion by HB11 avian macrophage cell line, and zymography confirming the presence of MMP2 in the avian vitreous humor (Takeyama et al., 2010; Webster and Crowe, 2006; Zhou et al., 2014). It is no surprise then that the NFL has elevated levels of gelatinase activity with potential sources of MMP2 originating from oligodendrocytes and vitreous humor macrophages.

Reduction of gelatinase activity in response to NMDA damage

In vitro experiments of extracted retinas indicated that there is a consistent and reproducible decrease in gelatinase activity after NMDA damage. This decrease in activity was sustained for several days after the initial insult, but returned to normal levels after seven days. This result was consistent with metabolic and mass normalization methods, reducing the possibility that differences were a result of damage-induced metabolic changes. These results were contrary to initial expectations due to the correlation of elevated MMP2 during ECM remodeling and damage repair

(Fawcett and Asher, 1999). We conducted follow-up experiments to understand the origins of this effect, and determine whether the effect may be related to a regenerative ECM microenvironment.

By using *in situ* gelatinase activity assays, we initially quantified no change in total activity across retinas treated with saline or NMDA. However, measurements of gelatinase activity within retinal layers revealed changes. Increases of gelatinase activity within the IPL correlated with decreases in TIMP2 distribution after NMDA damage. The scRNA-seq data indicate an increase in expression of TIMP2 from Müller glia, suggesting that Müller glia may underlie reduced in gelatinase activity in the IPL by providing inhibitor, TIMP2.

Alternatively, microglia in damaged retinas may mediate decreases in gelatinase activity. Microglia are commonly the mediator of neuroinflammation, and gelatinases such as MMP2 can activate pro-inflammatory cytokines such as IL-1β (Könnecke and Bechmann, 2013). Furthermore, microglia and inflammatory cytokines have been implicated as important mediators of neurogenesis in development as well as regeneration in the retina (Aguzzi et al., 2013; Fischer et al., 2014b; Sato, 2015). Therefore, we compared changes in gelatinase activity in microglia ablated retinas before and after NMDA damage. When comparing gelatinase activity after microglial ablation in the absence of NMDA damage, there is a notable decrease in enzyme activity. This suggests that microglia are playing a role in regulating gelatinases in the retina under homeostatic conditions, and that ablation reduces their global retinal activity. It should be noted that the standardization method impacted this analysis, as changes in gelatinase activity was not observed when microglia was ablated and standardized to metabolic activity. We interpret this difference to be due to microglial cell death reducing the average metabolic activity, which overestimates the gelatinase activity for a retinal tissue segment.

Then, we looked at the role of microglia influence on gelatinase activity with NMDA damage. Without affecting microglia, NMDA damage causes a significant decrease in gelatinase activity. When repeating the damage paradigm after microglia have been ablated, NMDA damage does not replicate this inhibitory effect on gelatinase activity. This implies that microglia are in part, directly or indirectly, involved in the down regulation of gelatinase activity after damage. Potential direct mechanisms include the secretion of MMPs, their proteolytic activators, or their associated inhibitors. Alternatively, an indirect mechanism to influence gelatinase activity would be the secretion of cytokines binding to cytokine receptors found on glia or neurons to induce gelatinases or their modulators. The scRNA seq suggested that microglia play a role in upregulating the production of TIMP3 in NIRGs after NMDA damage.

In the context of retinal damage and regeneration, findings indicate that an initiating inflammatory signal is required to initiate the process of reprogramming MG into MGPCs in zebrafish (Nelson et al., 2013b) and chick models (Fischer et al., 2014b). By contrast, sustained pro-inflammatory signaling may suppress the reprogramming of Müller glia and favor a gliotic, activated phenotype (Sifuentes et al., 2016; Widera et al., 2008). Tight coordination of these inflammatory signals may prove crucial for initial reprogramming and maintaining regeneration competency in the retina.

MMP2 enzymatic flux influence on MG reprogramming

When measuring global gelatinase activity with *in vitro* techniques of retinal tissue, there is a sustained decrease for several days after NMDA damage. This decrease appears to start several hours after NMDA damage and remains depressed for days. After 72 hrs the activity returns to normal and the GCL layer appears to increase in gelatinase activity according to in situ comparisons—further implicating oligodendrocytes as an origin of MMP2 secretion. When the gelatinase reduction is facilitated with different MMP2 inhibitors, we observe an increase in Edu$^+$ MGPCs. This result suggests that reducing gelatinase activity supports a regenerative microenvironment for de-differentiation into MGPCs.

In zebrafish, increasing MMP activity has been shown to increase proliferation in response to damage. Pan-MMP inhibitor GM6001 reduced proliferation, which was overcome by the administration of epidermal growth factor (EGF), suggesting that the EGF/EGFR pathway was dependent of MMP activity for reprogramming (Wan et al., 2012). The expression of MMP-9 increased the expression of transcription factor ASCL1a (Achaete-scute homolog 1) as determined through ASCLA1a luciferase assays and morpholino treatments (Kaur et al., 2018). These results indicate that MMP2 and MMP-9 may have different biological functions, or that the role of gelatinases in regeneration is variable among species.

In mammals, many paradigms of damage are associated with corresponding microglia activation and MMP secretion (Rosenberg, 2002). In these model species, there is limited regenerative responses to damage, and the predominant response is to generate a glial scar (Fawcett and Asher, 1999). Within the CNS, there is an upregulation of scarring factors from glia such as tenascin, brevican, neurocan, NG2,

TGFβ, and others (Fawcett and Asher, 1999; Penn et al., 2012). TGFβ is secreted into the ECM as a tripartite complex that permits the cytokine to remain latent and inactive until matrix degradation frees the protein for binding to the TGFβ receptor (Horiguchi et al., 2012). Previously, our lab and others have demonstrated that intraocular injection of TGFβ reduce MGPC proliferation through Smad 2/3 signaling (Close et al., 2006; Todd et al., 2017). Given the complex relationship of TGFβ with the ECM, the potential of this signaling cascade to be modulated by gelatinase activity present. Thus, we hypothesize that TGFβ may be one of the factors affected by reduced gelatinase activity to promote a regenerative response.

Dynamic changes of TIMP2 localization with NMDA damage

TIMP2 is a glycoprotein that is an endogenous inhibitor of MMPs, with increased specificity toward MMP2 (Nagase et al., 2006). Provided that MMP2 is the predominant gelatinase in the retina, and its activity decreases in response to NMDA damage, TIMP2 is a logical target to mediate this response. However, the relationship between MMP2 and TIMP2 is complicated by its noncanonical functions. TIMP2 can complex with MMP14 on the cell surface and activate pro-MMP2 (Emmert-Buck et al., 1995; Zucker et al., 1998). Some research suggests that TIMP2-MMP2 complex is the most efficient means of MMP2 activation *in vivo* (Wang et al., 2000). Furthermore, TIMP2 has been implicated in cytoplasmic functions independent of its effect on MMP2. In PC12 cells, increased TIMP2 increased p21^{cip}, decreased expression of cyclin B and D, and promoted neuronal differentiation through a cAMP/Rap1/ERK (Pérez-Martínez and Jaworski, 2005).

Our data suggests that TIMP2 is expressed predominantly by MG, but protein localization is found at higher concentration on the processes of bipolar cells. With NMDA damage, there is a dramatic decrease in TIMP2 only hours later in the IPL. Drastic changes in TIMP2 IPL localization imposed the question whether these changes were due to cell death, or dynamic trafficking and degradation of TIMP2. Previous data characterizing NMDA excitotoxicity on avian retina suggest that only a small fraction of bipolar cells die (Fischer et al., 1998). With this data in mind, our current hypothesis is that TIMP2 is being trafficked and localized differently in response to damage. However, PKCα did not remain a reliable marker of bipolar cell processes several days after damage, hence we cannot confidently conclude whether there was also robust remodeling of bipolar cell processes that coincide with TIMP2 changes.

In response, MG appear to upregulate TIMP2 expression and results in the partial restoration of the physiologic staining after 72 hours. The concurrent decrease in TIMP2 and decrease in MMP2 activity in the IPL occur during similar timeframes, leading to the hypothesis that TIMP2 may be playing a more significant role in MMP2 activation than inhibition in this context. Exogenous addition of TIMP2 after NMDA damage inhibits gelatinase activity, demonstrating behavior opposite of MMP2 inhibitors. Cell surface MMPs were detected on bipolar cells in the single cell sequencing data, suggesting the possibility that TIMP2 is complexed on the cell surface that serves as a cofactor in the proteolytic activation of gelatinases. The relatively low activity of gelatinases in the IPL may be due to other inhibitors, such as TIMP3 produced by NIRG cells also present in the IPL. Further investigation on the potential role of TIMP2 production by MG and localization on rod bipolar cells are required to understand the mechanism of gelatinase regulation after NMDA damage due to the diverse functions of TIMP2.

Conclusions

Gelatinases are known to play important roles regulating the ECM, including the development and physiologic function of retinal tissue. By using a combination of *in situ* zymography and *in vitro* tissue encapsulation techniques we quantified gelatinase activity after NMDA damage during MG reprogramming in the avian retina. Global retinal gelatinase activity significantly decreased after damage during the early reprogramming phase of MG with *in vitro* experiments. *In situ* experiments indicated significant decreases in IPL gelatinase activity which correlated with changes in TIMP2 and TIMP3 expression. Microglia were found to regulate MMP activity after damage, such as mediating an increase in TIMP3 mRNA in NIRG cells. Inhibition of gelatinase activity in retinas prior to an insult or growth factor treatment enhanced the formation of proliferating MGPCs. Inhibitors with specificity for MMP2, but not MMP-9, suppressed the formation of MGPCs. These findings are consistent with scRNA-seq transcriptomic data indicating that glial MMP2 is the primary gelatinase of the retina. These results emphasize the importance of gelatinase-mediated remodeling of ECM in cellular reprogramming, and may implicate different ECM-dependent growth factors that can impact MG and their regenerative potential.

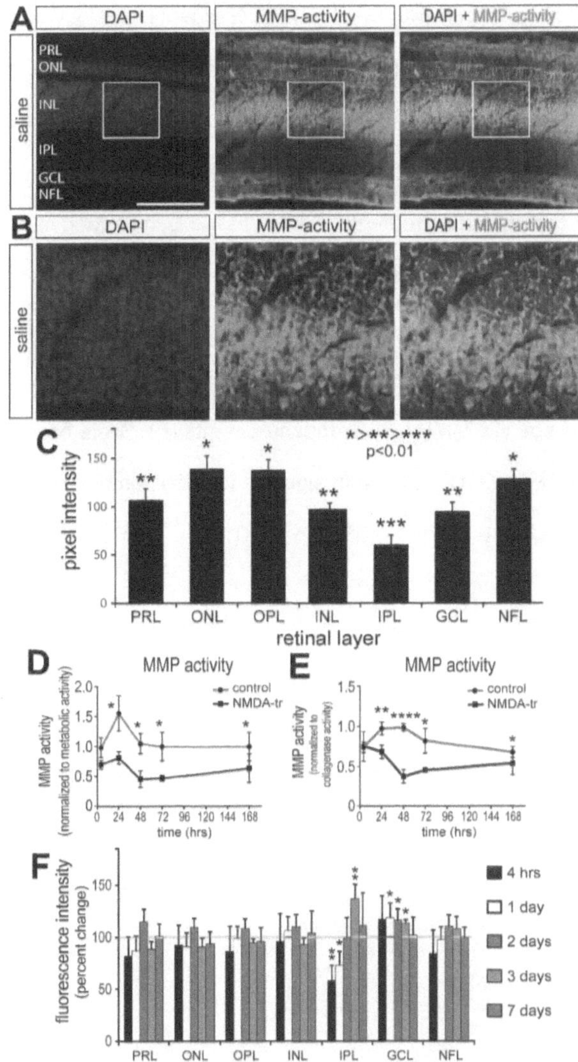

Figure 2.1. Gelatinase activity decreases in the retina after NMDA damage. Sections of normal, untreated retinas were incubated with DQ-gelatin which fluoresces when cleaved by MMP2/9 (**A**). Within the INL is a bistratified layer of MMP activity observed

paracellularly when costained with DAPI (**B**). Fluorescent intensity was quantified via densitometry to compare relative gelatinase activity (**C**) (n = 20). For simplicity, intensity is ranked with *>**>*** where p < 0.01 (**C**). Gelatinase activity was measured at various time points after NMDA-treatment. Each retina was horizontally hemisected for *in vitro* and *in situ* MMP activity measurements. Retinal tissue is imbedded in a hydrogel containing MMP 2/9 sensitive fluorescent peptides and normalized to metabolic activity (**D**) or collagenase activity (**E**) for direct comparison with tissue from saline vehicle injected eyes (n = 4). The remaining retina is cryo-sectioned and incubated in DQ peptide for region specific MMP activity measurements (**F**). Scale bar = 50μm. Error bars ± 1 SE (**F**) or ± 1 SD (**C**, **D**, **E**), with significance of difference determined by one-way ANOVA and Tukey test. * p < 0.05, ** p < 0.01 *** p < 0.001, **** p < 0.0001.

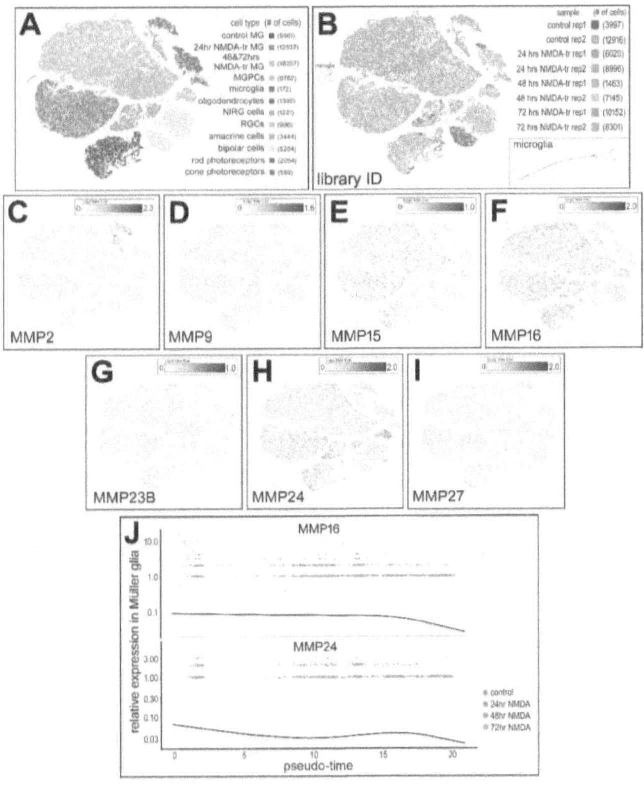

Figure 2.2 Patterns of MMP and TIMP expression in the avian retina after NMDA

damage. ScRNA-seq is used to identify gene expression in acutely dissociated retinal

cells. Two replicates are taken from control retinas (rep-1 3997 cells, rep-2 12916 cells)

and 24hrs (rep-1 6020 cells, rep-2 8996 cells), 48 hrs (rep-1 1463 cells, rep-2 7145

cells), and 72 hrs (rep-1 10152 cells, rep-2 8301 cells) after NMDA damage (**A**). tSNE

plots reduce the dimensionality of the data and organizes unbiased clusters on global

gene expression. Cluster identity is determined by hallmark gene expression. Microglia

(172 cells), rods (2054 cells), cones (589 cells), oligodendrocytes (1305 cells), Non-

astrocytic inner retinal glia (NIRG) (1221 cells), amacrine cells (3444 cells), bipolar cells (5254 cells), Müller glia (36588 cells), and Müller glia derived progenitors (6762 cells) are identified in these clusters (**B**). Müller glia were identified by collective expression of *LHX2, SOX9, RLBP1*, and *SLC1A3*. Oligodendrocytes were identified by *FGFR2, TGFB3, OLIG2, SOX10*. NIRGs are identified and differentiated from oligodendrocytes by *NKX2.2, PTPRZ1, SIX6*. In this scRNA library, heatmap panels are presented demonstrating MMP2 (**C**), MMP9 (**D**), MMP15 (**E**), MMP16 (**F**), MMP23B (**G**), MMP24 (**H**), and MMP27 (**I**) expression. Each dot is a cell where the color is a heat map with yellow = low expression, deep red = high expression, and grey = no expression. MMP16 and MMP24 expression is tracked across pseudotime in MG (**J**). Pseudotime represents the transition of MG to MGPCs after NMDA damage. The pseudotime trajectory was established for pseudotime states of different groups of variable genes, thereby establish a trajectory of resting Muller glia (high levels of mature glial markers, low levels of MGPC markers) to the left, and MGPCs (low levels of mature glial markers, high levels of MGPC markers) to the right.

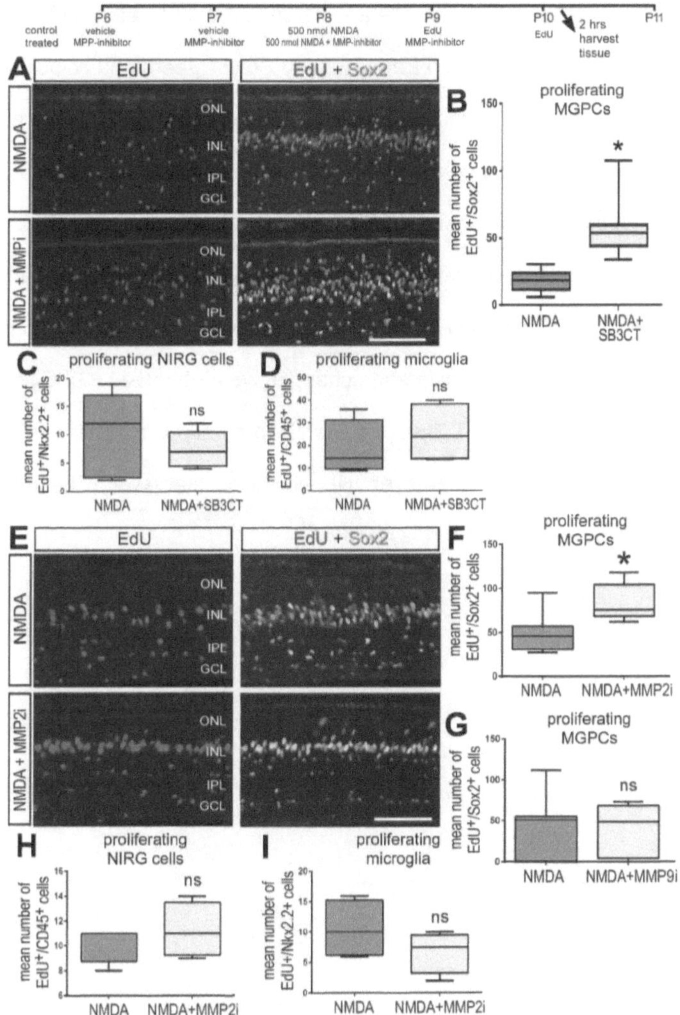

Figure 2.3. Gelatinase inhibitors SB-3CT and MMP2i II increase Müller glia proliferation

after NMDA damage. Avian retinas are injected intravitreally with a combination of

NMDA and SB-3CT (**A**). Retinas with MMP inhibitor treatment are given inhibitor injections 2 days prior to NMDA damage and harvested 2 days after NMDA damage. Retinal sections are co-labeled with Edu (red) and Sox2 (green) and colocalize on Müller glia derived progenitors and quantified (**B**). Proliferation of NIRG (**C**) and microglia (**D**) are quantified by colocalization of Edu and NKX 2.2 and CD45 respectively. The experimental paradigm was replicated with MMP 2i II (**E**) and Müller glia, NIRG, and microglia proliferation was quantified by colocalization of Edu (red) and Sox2 (green, **F**), NKX2.2 (**H**), and CD45 (**I**) respectively. When injected with the MMP-9 specific inhibitor (MMP-9i), no proliferation changes were observed (**G**). Significance was determined by a Student's T Test (n = 6) with *p < 0.05. Error bars are ± 1 SD. Abbreviations: ONL – outer nuclear layer, INL – inner nuclear layer, IPL – inner plexiform layer, GCL – ganglion cell layer.

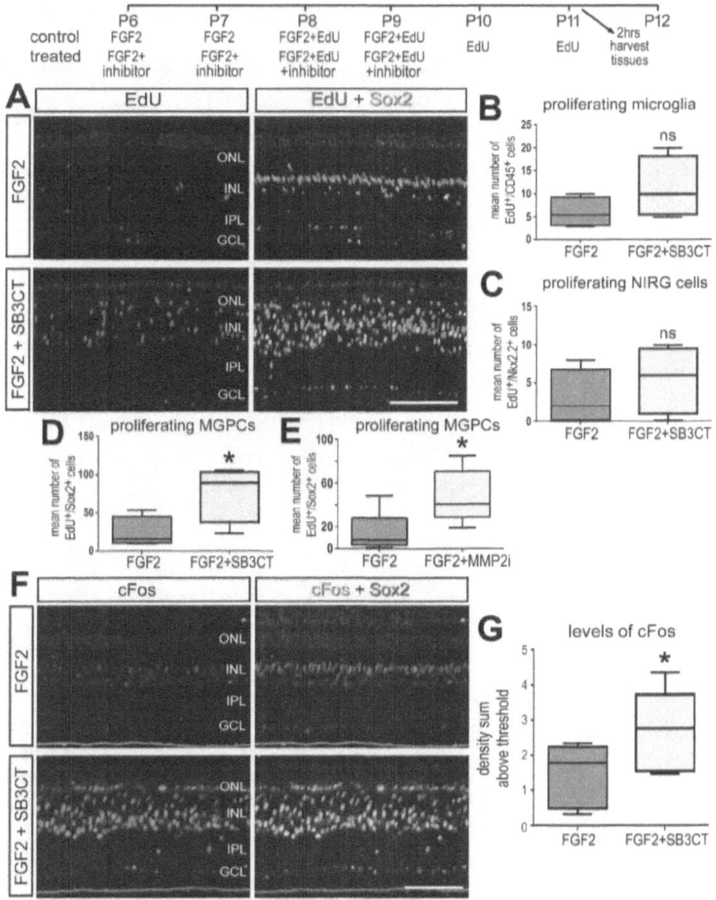

Figure 2.4. Gelatinase inhibitors SB-3CT and MMP2i II increase Müller glia proliferation

after FGF2 treatment. Avian retinas were injected intravitreally with a combination of

FGF2 and SB-3CT or MMP2i II over 4 days (**A**). Retinal sections are labeled with Edu

(red) and Sox2 (green) and colocalize on Müller glia derived progenitors. The number of

progenitors in a fixed area of the retina are counted and quantified (**B, C**). Proliferation

of microglia (**D**) and NIRG (**E**) are quantified by colocalization of Edu and NKX 2.2 and

CD45 respectively. cFos signaling with FGF2 and SB-3CT treatment was measured by colocalization of cFos (green) and Sox2(red) in nuclei (**E**). The density intensity sum in Sox2$^+$ nuclei is quantified (**F**). Significance was determined by a Student's T Test (n = 6) with *p < 0.05. Error bars are ± 1 SD. Abbreviations: ONL – outer nuclear layer, INL – inner nuclear layer, IPL – inner plexiform layer, GCL – ganglion cell layer.

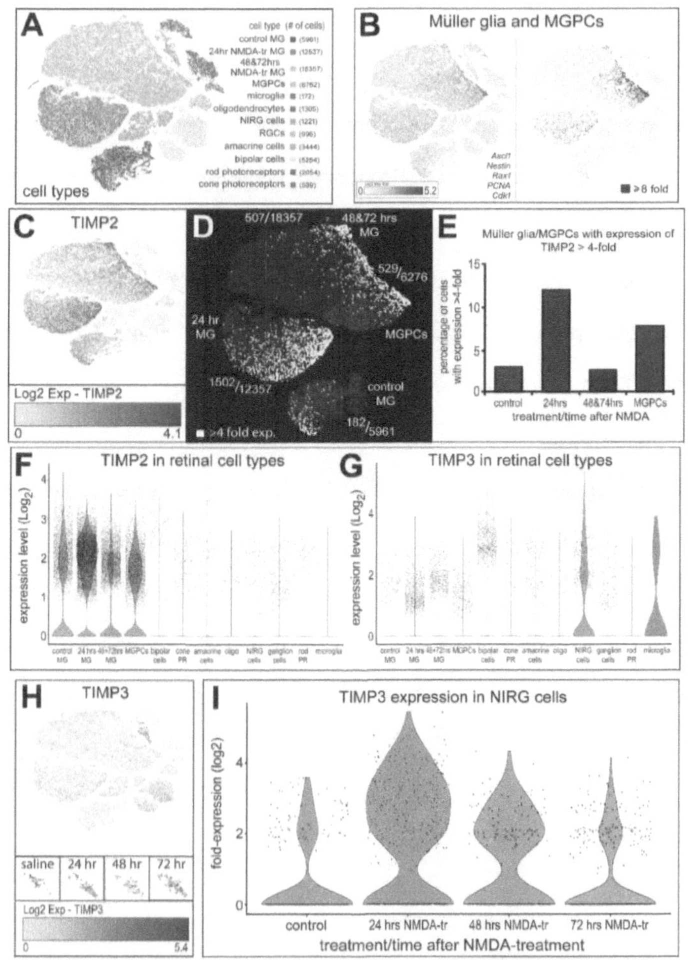

Figure 2.5 Müller glia and NIRGs secrete TIMPs in response to NMDA damage. Sc-RNA was used to identify gene expression in acutely dissociated retinal cells. tSNE plots reduce the dimensionality of the data and organizes unbiased clusters on global gene expression. Cluster identity are identified by hallmark gene expression. Microglia (172 cells), rods (2054 cells), cones (589 cells), oligodendrocytes (1305 cells), Non-

astrocytic inner retinal glia (NIRG) (1221 cells), amacrine cells (3444 cells), bipolar cells (5254 cells), Müller glia (36588 cells), and Müller glia derived progenitors (6762 cells) were identified in these clusters (A). Müller Glia were identified by collective expression of LHX2, SOX9, RLBP1, and Slc1a3. Progenitors were segregated to its own cluster by collective expression of Ascl1, Nestin, Rax1, PCNA, and Cdk1 (B). TIMP2 expression in Müller glia is represented on a heat map (C), with RNA levels ranging from 0 to ~17-fold over bassline reads per cell. Cells with transcriptional levels >4-fold are highlighted in each cluster (D) and the relative population of TIMP2 overexpression was quantified (E). TIMP3 expression is shown in the tSNE heat map (F), with expression ranging from 0 to ~42-fold over baselines reads per cell. Oligodendrocytes were identified by FGFR2, TGFB3, OLIG2, SOX10. NIRGs are identified and differentiated from oligodendrocytes by Nkx2.2, PTPRZ1, Six6. The NIRG clusters overlap significantly with control and treatment groups, and are separated to show relative TIMP3 expression at each time point. NIRG populations expressing $>\log_2(x)$ expression are quantified (G).

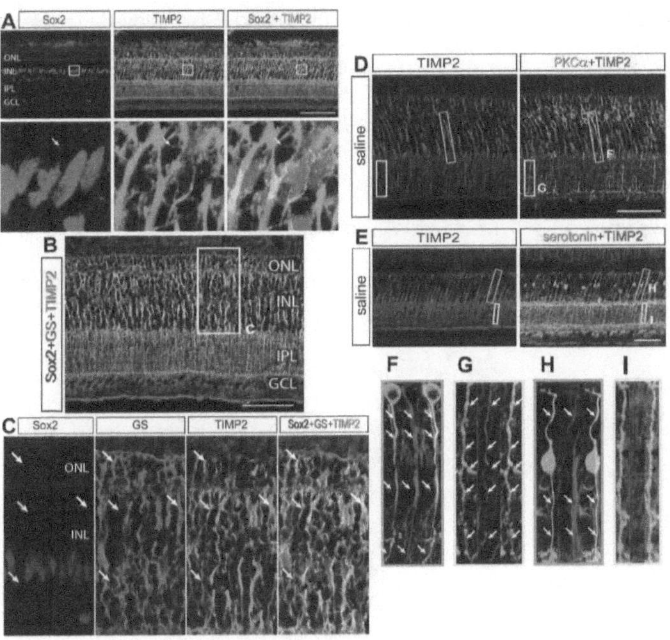

Figure 2.6. TIMP2 colocalizes to the cell surface of MG and PKCα bipolar cells. The retina was co-stained with Sox2 (red) and TIMP2(green) differentiating MG from other cell bodies in the INL (**A**). A portion of the retinal section is enlarged within the white box below the image. The white arrow indicates a TIMP2$^+$ neuronal cell body with a Sox2$^-$ nucleus and TIMP2$^+$ axonal projection. TIMP2 expression in MG is identified with immunolabelling colocalization of Sox2 (blue), glutamine synthetase (GS, red), and TIMP2 (green) (**B**). A portion of the retinal section is enlarged within the white box below the image, with white arrows identifying GS colocalization with TIMP2 and the yellow arrows labeling TIMP2 absent of MG markers (**C**). To determine the neuronal subtype colocalized with TIMP2 in the INL and IPL that are not MG, bipolar populations were labeled. Rod bipolar cells were identified with PKCα (**D**) and a subset of cone bipolar

cells with serotonin (**E**). Regions of the INL (blue) and IPL (yellow) are selected to demonstrate TIMP2$^+$ overlap for PKCα (**F, G**) and serotonin (**H, I**). Fasciculations of bipolar cell axons in the INL stain positive for TIMP2, where only PKCα processes are positive for TIMP2 in the IPL. White arrows indicate regions of TIMP2$^+$ overlap, where yellow arrows show TIMP2$^-$ regions. Abbreviations: ONL – outer nuclear layer, INL – inner nuclear layer, IPL – inner plexiform layer, GCL – ganglion cell layer. Scale bar = 50μm.

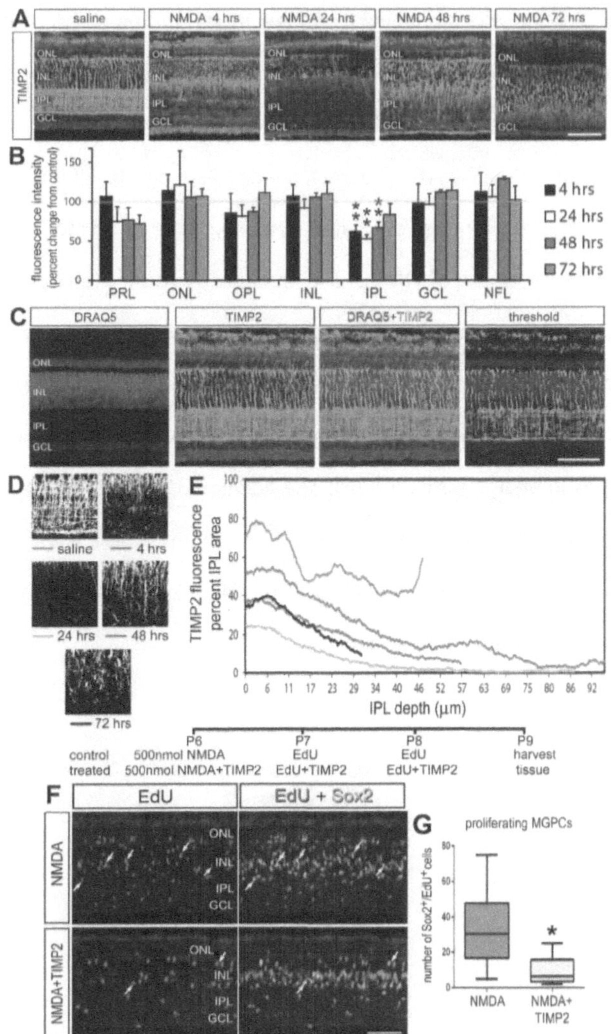

Figure 2.7. TIMP2 is redistributed in the IPL after damage and inhibits MGPC

formation. Retinas injected with NMDA are sectioned hours to days after damage (**A**).

Retinal sections are stained with TIMP2 with example images of each time point (n = 4).

The intensity of staining was quantified by densitometry and represented as a relative change to saline injected retinas (**B**). The change in TIMP2 distribution in the IPL is further quantified from hours to days following NMDA damage using DRAQ5 (red) and TIMP2 (green) immunolabeling (**C**). To track changes specific to TIMP2$^+$ processes in the IPL, a threshold filter removed any TIMP2 staining non-specific to neuronal processes. The average area of TIMP2$^+$ IPL processes is quantified from the inner INL border to the outer GCL border. The average area occupied by TIMP2$^+$ processes was calculated for each pixel (1 pixel = 0.29μm) in the IPL (**D, E**). Exogenous TIMP2 was injected intravitreally after NMDA damage to maintain elevated TIMP2 levels and measure changes in MGPC formation (**F**). The addition of TIMP2 inhibited the formation of MGPCs as measured by Sox2$^+$ Edu$^+$ nuclei (n = 12). Error bars are ± 1 SD. Scale bar = 50μm Abbreviations: ONL – outer nuclear layer, INL – inner nuclear layer, IPL – inner plexiform layer, GCL – ganglion cell layer.

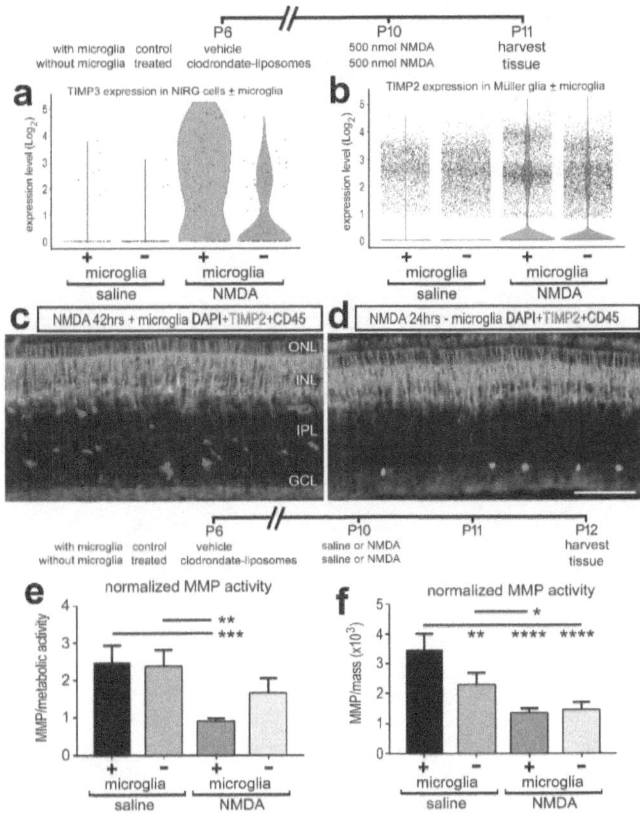

Figure 2.8. Microglia inhibit gelatinase activity after NMDA damage and promote the mRNA production of TIMP3 from NIRG cells. Microglia were ablated with clodronate liposomes and observed 24hrs after NMDA damage. Single cell sequencing detected a decrease in TIMP3 in NIRG cells in damaged retinas lacking microglia (**A**). TIMP2 protein distribution changes or mRNA levels in MG were unaffected by the loss of retinal microglia (n = 3) (**B, C, D**). Changes in gelatinase activity was measured with retinal tissue *in vitro* quantifications. Activity was normalized to metabolic activity (**E**) and mass

(**F**). (n = 4) for all experiments. The gelatinase activity of samples standardized for mass (**B, F**) were then normalized to the gelatinase activity a fixed concentration of collagenase. Error bars ± 1 SD, with significance of difference determined by one-way ANOVA and Tukey's post-test. * $p < 0.05$, ** $p < 0.01$ *** $p < 0.001$, **** $p < 0.0001$.

Chapter 3

Midkine is neuroprotective and influences glial reactivity and the formation of Müller glia-derived progenitor cells in chick and mouse retinas

Introduction

Midkine (MDK) and pleiotrophin (PTN) are secreted factors that belong to a family of basic heparin-binding cytokines (Muramatsu, 2002). The C-terminal domain of MDK interacts with carbohydrate-bindings proteins which facilitate dimerization and cell signaling (Fabri et al., 1993; Iwasaki et al., 1997; Kilpeläinen et al., 2000; Tsutsui et al., 1991). Extracellular matrix proteoglycans that have a high binding-affinity for MDK include protein tyrosine phosphatase-ζ receptor-like 1 (PTPRZ1), syndecans, glypican-2, PG-M/versican, integrin $\alpha_6\beta_1$, low density lipoprotein receptor-related protein (LRP), and neuroglycans (Ichihara-Tanaka et al., 2006; Kojima et al., 1996; Kurosawa et al., 2001; Maeda et al., 1999; Mitsiadis et al., 1995; Muramatsu et al., 2000; Muramatsu et al., 2004; Nakanishi et al., 1997; Zou et al., 2000). MDK forms a complex with these proteoglycans to initiate cell-signaling through receptor tyrosine kinases and activation of second messengers such as src, PI-3K, and PAK1 (Qi et al., 2001; Shen et al., 2015; Thillai et al., 2016).

During development the roles of MDK are conserved across many vertebrate species including fish, mice, and humans (Tsutsui et al., 1991). MDK has different functions including promoting cell survival and proliferation, acting directly on stem cells during normal fetal development and organogenesis (Mitsiadis et al., 1995). MDK has been implicated in the pathogenesis of more than 20 different types of cancers, resistance to chemotherapeutics, increased survival of cancerous cells with acidosis and hypoxia, and elevated levels of MDK have been correlated with poor prognoses (Dai et al., 2009; Kang et al., 2004; Mashima et al., 2009; Mirkin et al., 2005; Reynolds et al., 2004; Salama et al., 2006; Takei et al., 2001; Takei et al., 2006; Tsutsui et al., 1993). In the damaged mammalian CNS, MDK expression is elevated and may support neuronal survival (Jochheim-Richter et al., 2006; Kikuchi-Horie et al., 2004; Miyashiro et al., 1998; Obama et al., 1998; Sakakima et al., 2006). In rodent eyes, subretinal delivery of MDK protects photoreceptors from light-mediated degeneration (Unoki et al., 1994). In sum, MDK has pleiotropic functions that are context dependent.

In fish, retinal regeneration is a robust process that restores neurons and visual function following damage, whereas this process is far less robust in birds and nearly absent in mammals (Hitchcock and Raymond, 1992; Karl et al., 2008; Raymond, 1991). Müller glia (MG) have been identified as the cell-of-origin for progenitors in mature retinas (Bernardos et al., 2007; Fausett and Goldman, 2006; Fausett et al., 2008; Fischer and Reh, 2001; Ooto et al., 2004). Mammalian retina requires significant stimulation, such as forced expression of Ascl1, inhibition of histone deacetylases, and neuronal damage to reprogram MG into progenitor-like cells (Karl et al., 2008; Pollak et al., 2013b, 1; Ueki et al., 2015). In the chick retina, MG readily reprogram into progenitor-like cells that proliferate, but the progeny have a limited capacity to differentiate as neurons (Fischer and Reh, 2001; Fischer and Reh, 2003). Understanding the mechanisms that regulate the proliferation and differentiation of

MGPCs is important to harnessing the regenerative potential of MG in warm-blooded vertebrates.

Recent studies in the zebrafish retina have indicated that MDK-a is upregulated in stem cell niches and by MG during reprogramming into neurogenic progenitor cells (Calinescu et al., 2009). MDK-a is expressed by mitotic retinal progenitors at 30 hrs post-fertilization, then in differentiating MG at 72 hrs post-fertilization and expression is maintained in mature MG (Gramage et al., 2014). During reprogramming of MG into MGPCs, MDK-a regulates cell cycle progression and influences retinal development through the HLH transcription factor Id2a (Luo et al., 2012; Nagashima et al., 2019b). Although PTN is expressed by retinal progenitors during mammalian development, its expression has been correlated with cell cycle exit and differentiation of neurons and glia (Hienola et al., 2004; Jung et al., 2004; Roger et al., 2006). Nothing is known about how MDK influences the process of retinal regeneration in warm-blooded vertebrates. Accordingly, we investigated expression pattern and function of MDK and PTN on glial cells in the chick and mouse retinas *in vivo*.

Methods and Materials:

Animals:

The use of animals was in accordance with the guidelines established by the National Institutes of Health and IACUC at The Ohio State University. Newly hatched P0 wildtype leghorn chicks (*Gallus gallus domesticus*) were obtained from Meyer Hatchery (Polk, Ohio). Post-hatch chicks were maintained in a regular diurnal cycle of 12 hours light, 12 hours dark (8:00 AM-8:00 PM). Chicks were housed in stainless-steel brooders at 25°C and received water and Purina[tm] chick starter *ad libitum*. Mice were kept on a cycle of 12 h light, 12 h dark (lights on at 6:00 AM). C57BL/6J mice between the ages of P60-P100 were used for all experiments.

Fertilized eggs were obtained from the Michigan State University, Department of Animal Science. Eggs were incubated at a constant 37.5°C, with a 1hr period room temperature cool down every 24hrs. Additionally, the eggs were rocked every 45 minutes, and held at a constant relative humidity of 45%. Embryos were harvested at various time points after incubation and staged according to guidelines established by Hamburger and Hamilton ((Hamburger, 1951)).

Intraocular injections:

Chicks were anesthetized with 2.5% isoflurane mixed with oxygen from a non-rebreathing vaporizer. The technical procedures for intraocular injections were performed as previously described (Fischer et al., 1998). With all injection paradigms, both pharmacological and vehicle treatments were administered to the right and left eye respectively at the same time of day for consecutive daily injections. Drugs were injected in 20 ml of 30% DMSO or sterile saline with 0.05 mg/ml bovine serum albumin added as a carrier. For mice injections, the total volume injected into each eye was 2µl. The specific details of the injected compounds are described (Table S1). Schematic figures for treatment paradigms indicate the days of drug delivery for each eye and are included for each dataset in figures.

Single Cell RNA sequencing

Retinas were obtained from embryonic, postnatal chick, and adult mouse retinas.
Isolated retinas were dissociated in a 0.25% papain solution in Hank's balanced salt
solution (HBSS), pH = 7.4, for 30 minutes, and suspensions were frequently triturated.
The dissociated cells were passed through a sterile 70μm filter to remove large
particulate debris. Dissociated cells were assessed for viability (Countess II; Invitrogen)
and cell-density diluted to 700 cell/μl. Each single cell cDNA library was prepared for a
target of 10,000 cells per sample. The cell suspension and Chromium Single Cell 3' V2
reagents (10X Genomics) were loaded onto chips to capture individual cells with
individual gel beads in emulsion (GEMs) using 10X Chromium Controller. cDNA and
library amplification for an optimal signal was 12 and 10 cycles respectively.
Sequencing was conducted on Illumina HiSeq2500 (Genomics Resource Core Facility,
John's Hopkins University) or HiSeq4000 (Novogene) with 26 bp for Read 1 and 98 bp
for Read 2. Fasta sequence files were de-multiplexed, aligned, and annotated using the
chick ENSMBL database (GRCg6a, Ensembl release 94) or mouse ENSMBL database
(GRCm38.p6, Ensembl release 67) by using Cell Ranger software. Gene expression
was counted using unique molecular identifier bar codes, and gene-cell matrices were
constructed. Using Seurat toolkits, t-distributed stochastic neighbor embedding (tSNE)
plots or Uniform Manifold Approximation and Projection for Dimension Reduction
(UMAP) plots were generated from aggregates of multiple scRNA-seq libraries (Butler
et al., 2018; Satija et al., 2015). Compiled in each tSNE/UMAP plot are two biological
library replicates for each experimental condition. Seurat was used to construct
violin/scatter plots. Significance of difference in violin/scatter plots was determined using
a Wilcoxon Rank Sum test with Bonferroni correction. Monocle was used to construct

unbiased pseudo-time trajectories and scatter plotters for MG and MGPCs across pseudotime (Qiu et al., 2017a; Qiu et al., 2017b; Trapnell et al., 2012). Genes that were used to identify different types of retinal cells included the following: (1) Müller glia: *GLUL, VIM, SCL1A3, RLBP1*, (2) MGPCs: *PCNA, CDK1, TOP2A, ASCL1*, (3) microglia: *C1QA, C1QB, CCL4, CSF1R, TMEM22*, (4) ganglion cells: *THY1, POU4F2, RBPMS2, NEFL, NEFM*, (5) amacrine cells: *ELAVL4, GAD67, CALB2, TFAP2A*, (6) horizontal cells: *PROX1, CALB2, NTRK1* (only in chick), (7) bipolar cells: *VSX1, OTX2, GRIK1, GABRA1*, and (7) cone photoreceptors: *CALB1* (only in chick), *GNAT2, OPN1LW*, and (8) rod photoreceptors: *RHO, NR2E3, ARR3*. The MG have an over-abundant representation in the scRNA-seq databases. This likely resulted from fortuitous capture-bias and/or tolerance of the MG to the dissociation process. Single cell libraries for NMDA and FGF insulin in the mouse and chick generated by our lab have first been reported for cross species comparisons (Hoang et al., 2020), where chick embryonic retinal libraries are first being reported in this study.

Fixation, sectioning, and immunocytochemistry:

Retinal tissue samples were formaldehyde fixed, sectioned, and labeled via immunohistochemistry as described previously (Fischer et al., 2008; Fischer et al., 2009b). Antibody dilutions and commercial sources for images used in this study are described (Table S2). Observed labeling was not due to off-target labeling of secondary antibodies or tissue autofluorescence because sections incubated exclusively with secondary antibodies were devoid of fluorescence. Secondary antibodies utilized include donkey-anti-goat-Alexa488/568, goat-anti-rabbit-Alexa488/568/647, goat-anti-mouse-Alexa488/568/647, goat-anti-rat-Alexa488 (Life Technologies) diluted to 1:1000 in PBS and 0.2% Triton X-100.

Fluorescent in situ hybridization (FISH):

The FISH protocol has been adapted from the hybridization chain reaction (HCR) for tissue sections provided by Molecular Instruments. Briefly, the retinal tissue was dissected and fixed in 4% PFA in DEPC water with 2mM EDTA for 4 hrs. Tissues were washed for 30 min in 0.1% Tween-20 PBS (PWT) and set overnight into 30% sucrose. Tissues were cryosectioned and retinal sections were rehydrated in PWT for 15 min on a shaker. Sections were moved to 2x SSCT for 20 minutes. Hybridization buffer was incubated on the slide at 37°C. The buffer was removed, and the probe-set diluted 1:50 in hybridization buffer was set to incubate in a humidified chamber at 37°C for 24 hrs. The probe was removed with wash buffer for 15 minutes at 37°C and 5x SSCT for 5 minutes at room temperature. The amplification primers were snap cooled, mixed, and applied to the sections at room temperature for 24hrs in the dark. The primers were washed off with 5x SSCT for 10 minutes, and glass cover slips mounted for imaging.

Labeling for EdU:

The incorporation of EdU into proliferating nuclei was detected using a copper-catalyzed reaction of 5-ethynyl-2'-deoxyuridine (Click-It Labeling Technology; Thermo Fisher Scientific) with an Azide fluorophore (Thermo Fisher Scientific) to form a stable triazole ring. For experiments where EdU was administered, immunolabeled sections were fixed in 4% formaldehyde in 0.1M PBS pH 7.4 for 5 minutes at room temperature.

Samples were washed for 5 minutes with PBS, permeabilized with 0.5% Triton X-100 in

PBS for 1 minute at room temperature and washed twice for 5 minutes in PBS. Sections

were incubated for 30 minutes at room temperature in a buffer consisting of 100 mM

Tris, 8 mM $CuSO_4$, and 100 mM ascorbic acid in dH_2O with an Alexa Fluor 568 Azide

(Thermo Fisher Scientific) added to the buffer at a 1:100 dilution.

Terminal deoxynucleotidyl transferase dUTP nick end labeling (TUNEL):

The TUNEL assay was implemented to identify dying cells by imaging

fluorescent labeling of double stranded DNA breaks in nuclei. The *In Situ* Cell Death Kit

(TMR red; Roche Applied Science) was applied to fixed retinal sections as per the

manufacturer's instructions.

Photography, measurements, cell counts and statistics:

Microscopy images of retinal sections were captured with the Leica DM5000B

microscope with epifluorescence and the Leica DC500 digital camera. High resolution

confocal images were obtained with a Leica SP8 available in The Department of

Neuroscience Imaging Facility at The Ohio State University. Representative images are

modified to have enhanced color, brightness, and contrast for improved clarity using

Adobe Photoshop. In EdU proliferation assays, a fixed region of retina was counted and

average numbers of Sox2 and EdU co-labeled cells. The retinal region selected for

investigation was standardized between treatment and control groups to reduce

variability and improve reproducibility.

Similar to previous reports (Fischer et al., 2009a; Fischer et al., 2009b; Ghai et al., 2009), immunofluorescence was quantified by using ImagePro6.2 (Media Cybernetics, Bethesda, MD, USA) or Image J (NIH). Identical illumination, microscope, and camera settings were used to obtain images for quantification. Retinal areas were sampled from 5.4 MP digital images. These areas were randomly sampled over the inner nuclear layer (INL) where the nuclei of the bipolar and amacrine neurons were observed. Measurements of immunofluorescence were performed using ImagePro 6.2 as described previously (Ghai et al., 2009; Stanke et al., 2010; Todd and Fischer, 2015). The density sum was calculated as the total of pixel values for all pixels within thresholded regions. The mean density sum was calculated for the pixels within threshold regions from ≥5 retinas for each experimental condition. GraphPad Prism 6 was used for statistical analyses.

Measurement for immunofluorescence of cFos in the nuclei of MG/MGPCs were made by from single optical confocal sections by selecting the total area of pixel values above threshold (≥70) for Sox2 or Sox9 immunofluorescence (in the red channel) and copying nuclear cFos from only MG (in the green channel). The MG-specific cFos was quantified (as described below). Measurements of cFos or pS6 immunofluorescence were made for a fixed, cropped areas (14,000 μm^2) of INL, OPL and ONL. Measurements were made for regions containing pixels with intensity values of 70 or greater (0 = black and 255 = saturated). The intensity sum was calculated as the total of pixel values for all pixels within threshold regions. The mean intensity sum was calculated for the pixels within threshold regions from ≥5 retinas for each experimental condition.

To test for normality, we performed a Levine's test. For statistical evaluation of differences in treatments, a two-tailed paired *t*-test was applied to account for intra-individual variability where each biological sample provides a control. For two treatment groups comparing assessing significant across inter-individual variability, a two-tailed unpaired *t*-test was applied. For multivariate analysis, an ANOVA with the associated Tukey Test was used to evaluate any significant differences between multiple groups.

Results:

MDK and _PTN_ are upregulated in maturing MG during chick retinal development

scRNA-seq retina libraries were established at four stages of development including E5, E8, E12, and E15. The aggregation of these libraries yielded 22,698 cells after filtering to exclude doublets, cells with low UMI, and low genes/cell. UMAP plots of aggregate libraries of embryonic retinas formed clustered of cells into patterns that correlated to both developmental stage and cell type (Fig. 3.1a). Cell types were identified based on expression of well-established markers. Specifically, retinal progenitor cells from E5 and E8 retinas were identified by expression of *ASCL1, CDK1,* and *TOP2A.* (Fig. 3.12a,b). Maturing MG were identified by expression of *GLUL, RLBP1* and *SLC1A3* (Fig. 3.12a,b).

Elevated levels of *MDK* expression were observed in MG at E12 and E15, with lower levels of expression in immature MG at E8 and retinal progenitor cells at E5 (Fig. 3.1c,d). *PTN* was prominently expressed in immature and mature MG, but was also detected in immature amacrine cells (E8), rod photoreceptors (E12), and cone photoreceptors (E15) (Fig. 3.1c). Levels of *MDK* and *PTN* were significantly higher in maturing MG compared to immature MG and RPCs (Fig. 3.1d). Putative receptors and signal transducers of MDK and PTN include integrin β1 (*ITGB1*), receptor-like protein tyrosine phosphatase-ζ (*PTPRZ1*), chondroitin sulfate proteoglycan 5 (*CSPG5*) and p21-activated serine/threonine kinase (*PAK1*). These mRNAs had variable, low levels of expression in embryonic retinal cells. *PTPRZ1*, *ITGB1* and *PAK1* were observed in RPCs, immature and mature MG (Fig. 3.12c). *CSPG5* was expressed by developing photoreceptors, amacrine, ganglion and bipolar cells (Fig. 3.1c). Additionally, *CSPG5* was expressed at elevated levels by immature and maturing MG compared to levels see in RPCs (Fig. 3.1c.d). We did not detect expression of anaplastic lymphoma kinase (*ALK*; ENSGALG00000009034), a putative receptor for MDK and PTN (Stoica et al., 2001) in any type of cell in embryonic or mature chick retina.

Re-embedding of RPCs and MG for pseudotime analysis revealed an ordering of cells with early RPCs and maturing MG at opposite ends of the trajectory (Fig. 3.1e). Across the pseudotime trajectory levels of *GLUL* increased, while levels of *CDK1* decreased (Fig. 3.12e,f). Similar to the pattern of expression of *GLUL*, the expression of *MDK* and *PTN* increases from retinal progenitors to maturing MG (Fig. 3.1e,f). Higher levels of expression were observed for both *MDK* and *PTN* in maturing MG, with *PTN* at low levels in retinal progenitors (Fig. 3.1f,g). Across pseudotime, levels of *MDK* were high in early progenitors, with a dip in expression during transition phases, and increased in maturing MG (Fig. 3.1f,g). Collectively, these findings suggest that both *PTN* and *MDK* are upregulated by maturing MG during late stages of embryonic development, and, based on patterns of expression of putative receptors, MDK and PTN may have autocrine and paracrine actions in late-stage embryonic chick retinas.

MDK is upregulated in MG of damaged chick retinas

Chick retinas were damaged with NMDA, an established method of excitotoxic damage that rapidly induces neuronal death and can stimulate MG to de-differentiate and form proliferating MGPCs (Fischer and Reh, 2001). NMDA-induced retinal damage has been widely used to study to formation of MGPCs in the retinas of fish, chicks and rodents (Gallina et al., 2014a). Accordingly, we established scRNA-seq libraries for retinal cells at different times after NMDA-treatment (Hoang et al., 2020). These data were analyzed to assess levels of expression of *MDK, PTN* and putative down-stream signaling genes in retinal neurons and glia following a damage paradigm where MGPCs are formed.

scRNA-seq libraries were aggregated for retinal cells obtained from control and NMDA-damaged retinas respectively at various time points (24, 48 and 72 hrs) after treatment (Fig. 3.2a). UMAP plots were generated and clusters of different cells were identified based on well-established patterns of expression (Fig. 3.2a,b). For example, resting MG formed a discrete cluster of cells and expressed high levels of *GLUL, RLBP1* and *SLC1A3* (Fig. 3.13a,b). After damage, MG down-regulate markers of mature glia as they transition into reactive glial cells and into progenitor-like cells that up-regulate *TOP2A, CDK1* and *ESPL1* (Fig. 3.13a,b). *MDK* was expressed at low levels in few resting MG in undamaged retina, unlike maturing MG in late stages of embryonic retinas (Fig. 3.1c,e), suggesting a down-regulation of *MDK* in MG as development proceeds after hatching. *MDK* was detected in a few oligodendrocytes and Non-astrocytic Inner Retinal Glia (NIRGs). NIRG cells are a distinct type of glial cells that has been described in the retinas of birds (Fischer et al., 2010; Rompani and Cepko, 2010) and some types of reptiles (Todd et al., 2015). Following NMDA-induced damage, *MDK* is upregulated in MG and MGPCs at 24hrs, 48hrs, and 72hrs after treatment (Fig. 3.2c,e). In addition, MGPCs maintain high levels of *MDK* (Fig. 3.2c,e). By comparison, *PTN* was widely expressed in most types of retinal cells and was significantly downregulated by MG and MGPCs in damaged retinas (Fig. 2c,e). We queried expression of putative receptors for *MDK* and *PTN*, including *PTPRZ1, CSPG5* and Syndecan 4 (*SDC4*). Although *SDC4* was expressed in few retina cells, *SDC4* was low in resting MG and was upregulated across many MG at 24hrs after NMDA-treatment (Fig. 3.2d,e). *CSPG5* was expressed at high levels in resting MG and was downregulated in activated MG at 24hrs after NMDA and in MGPCs, and remained elevated in activated MG at 48 and 72hrs after NMDA (Fig. 3.2d,e). *PTPRZ1* was not detected in MG, but was expressed at high levels in NIRG cells and in a few amacrine and bipolar cells (Fig. 3.2d). *CSPG5, SDC4,* and *ITGB1* were dynamically expressed by different retinal neurons and NIRG cells in NMDA-damaged retinas (Fig. 3.13a-e), suggesting that MDK may influence NIRG cells and neurons following injury.

To validate some of the findings from scRNA-seq we performed fluorescence *in situ* hybridization (FISH) for *MDK* and *PTN*. FISH for *MDK* demonstrated no signal in undamaged retinas, whereas robust signal for *MDK* appeared in the INL at 24hrs after NMDA-treatment (Fig 3.2j). This signal co-localized with glutamine synthetase immunoreactivity in MG (Fig. 3.2k). In undamaged retinas, FISH for *PTN* revealed signal within the ONL (photoreceptors), cells in the distal INL (bipolar cells and MG), and a few scattered cells in IPL and GCL (putative NIRG cells) (Fig. 3.2j). In NMDA-damaged retinas, FISH for *PTN* appeared unchanged in the ONL, was diminished in the distal INL (damaged or dying bipolar cells), but appeared concentrated in the middle of the INL and overlapped with signal for MDK (Fig. 3.2j). The FISH for *MDK* and *PTN* closely match the patterns of expression from scRNA-seq within retinal cells.

We re-embedded scRNA-seq data to establish a pseudotime trajectory on these datasets to better assess changes in expression of MDK-related genes during the transition of MG to progenitor cells after damage (Fig. 3.14). Analysis of different pseudotime states revealed a branched trajectory with resting MG, proliferating MGPCs, and activated MG from 72hr after NMDA-treatment largely confined to different branches and states (Fig. 3.14a-d). The expression of *MDK* across pseudotime positively correlates with a transition toward an MGPC-phenotype and upregulation of progenitor markers, such as *CDK1*, and inversely correlated to resting glial phenotypes with significant down-regulation of glial markers such as *GLUL* (Fig. 3.14a-d). By comparison, levels of *PTN* were decreased across pseudotime, with the largest decrease in *PTN* in activated MG compared to resting MG (Fig. 3.14a-d). Similar to expression patterns of *CDK1*, patterns of expression of *SDC4* are significantly elevated in pseudotime state 4 populated by activated MG and proliferating MGPCs (Fig. 3.14a-d). In sum, these pseudotime trajectories showed similar patterns of expression for MDK and PTN as those seen in UMAP analyses in Fig 2e, with MDK increasing and PTN decreasing in activated MG and MGPCs after neuronal injury.

When comparing MG and MGPCs from 48hrs after NMDA with and without FGF2 and insulin, the relative levels of *MDK* and *PTN* were significantly decreased (Fig. 2f-i). UMAP plots revealed distinct clustering of MG and MGPCs from retinas from 48hrs

NMDA alone and 48hrs NMDA plus FGF2 and insulin (Fig. 3.2f-i). Similarly, levels of *GLUL, RLBP1* and *CSPG5* were significantly decreased by FGF2 and insulin in damaged retinas in both MG and MGPCs (Fig. 3.2f-l; Fig. 3.14e-g). By contrast, levels of *CDK1* and *TOP2A* were significantly increased by FGF2 and insulin in MGPCs in damaged retinas (Fig. 3.14e-g). Collectively, these findings suggest expression levels of *PTN* reflects a resting glial phenotype and levels are decreased by damage and further decreased by FGF2 and insulin. Expression levels of *MDK* corresponds with acutely activated glia, which is strongly induced by damage, but decreased by FGF2 and insulin in damaged retinas. Furthermore, because FGF2 and insulin are neuroprotective, it is possible that decreased upregulation of MDK, PTN and CSPG5 in MG result secondarily from reduced levels of neuronal death.

Exogenous MDK is neuroprotective and induces cFos and pS6 in chick MG

The large, significant upregulation of *MDK* by MG in NMDA-treated retinas suggests that this growth factor is involved in the responses of retinal cells to acute damage. To determine whether MDK influences retinal cells we probed for the activation of different cell-signaling pathways following a single intraocular injection of recombinant MDK or PTN. Chick recombinant MDK was utilized due to poor conservation between mouse and human homologs (48% and 42% respectively). Four hours after delivery of MDK we found a significant upregulation of cFos and pS6 specifically in MG (Fig. 3.3a-e), suggesting activation of the mTor-pathway. In addition, amacrine cells appeared to significantly up-regulate cFos and NIRG cells upregulated pS6 in response to MDK (Fig. 3.3a-e). To test whether cell signaling was influenced by

PP2A-inhibitors, we co-applied fostriecin and calyculin A with MDK. We found that fostriecin and calyculin A significantly reduced levels of pS6 in MDK-treated MG (Fig. 3.3f,g), where cFos activation was unaffected and independent of PP2A inhibition (data not shown). There were no detectable changes in levels of pERK1/2, p38 MAPK, pCREB, pSmad1/5/8, pStat3, and nuclear smad2/3 following intravitreal delivery of MDK. We did not detect changes in cell signaling in response to intraocular injections of PTN. Four consecutive daily intraocular injections of MDK or PTN had no significant effect upon MG reactivity or formation of proliferating MGPCs.

Injections of MDK after NMDA-treatment had no significant effect upon glial reactivity or proliferation of MGPCs, NIRG cells or microglia. Administration of MDK after NMDA lacked significant effects likely because endogenous levels of MDK were very high and MDK-mediated cell-signaling may have been saturated. By comparison, injection of MDK prior to NMDA-treatment significantly reduced the numbers of proliferating MGPCs that accumulated EdU or were immunolabeled for pHisH3 (Fig. 3.4a-d). We probed for changes in NIRG cells and microglia in the chick retina after damage, as both cell types are known to proliferation and transiently accumulate in the retina after damage (Zelinka et al., 2012). There was a significant reduction in the total number NIRG cells that accumulated in NMDA-damaged retinas (Fig. 3.4e,f). These cells were identified and quantified by $Sox2^+/Nkx2.2^+$ colocalization. In addition, microglial reactivity was influenced by MDK. We measured the area and intensity sum for CD45 immunofluorescence, which is known to be increased in reactive microglia (Fischer et al., 2014b). Both the area and the intensity of CD45-immunofluorescence was decreased in response to MDK (Fig. 3.4g,h). There were no detected MDK-mediated changes in read-outs of different cell-signaling pathways including pS6, pCREB, p38 MAPK, pERK1/2, or pStat3 after damage (data not shown).

Levels of retinal damage and cell death are known to positively correlate to numbers of proliferating MGPCs (Fischer and Reh, 2001; Fischer and Reh, 2003). Thus, it is possible that reduced numbers of proliferating MGPCs resulted from less cell death with MDK pre-treatment. Using the TUNEL method to label dying cells, we found that the administration of MDK before NMDA-damage significantly reduced numbers of dying cells (Fig. 3.4i,j). Decreased numbers of dying cells were observed at both 24h and 72h after NMDA-treatment with MDK pre-treatment. To complement the cell death studies, we probed for long-term survival of inner retinal neurons. NMDA damage results in death of amacrine and bipolar cells, and survival was measured by cell counts after cell death and clearance. Although there was no change in numbers of AP2α^{+} amacrine cells, there was a significantly increased number of surviving calretinin+ cells in retinas treated with MDK (Fig. 3.4k,i), indicating that MDK promoted the survival of subtypes of amacrine cells.

PTN was significantly downregulated in MG following NMDA-treatment (Fig. 2). Despite the administration of high doses (1μg/dose) of PTN, intravitreal delivery of PTN with NMDA had no measurable effects on the formation of MGPCs, the reactivity and proliferation of microglia, and accumulation of NIRG cells (data not shown). Although these experiments were conducted using recombinant human PTN, there is high conservation between chick, mouse and human PTN (92% and 93% respectively).

Inhibition of MDK-signaling increases cell death and reduces MGPC formation in chick

MDK-signaling is often upregulated in tissues with proliferating cells, such as tumors, and this proliferation can be suppressed by inhibition of MDK-signaling (Hao et al., 2013; Takei et al., 2006). Since levels of *MDK* were markedly increased in MG in damaged retinas, we tested whether inhibition of MDK-signaling depressed the formation of proliferating MGPCs. We applied a MDK-expression inhibitor (MDKi), which downregulates protein expression in a dose dependent manner (Masui et al., 2016). However, application of MDKi after NMDA-treatment did not influence MG, NIRG cells, or microglia (data not shown). Alternatively, we applied a PTPRZ inhibitor SCB4380 that targets the intracellular domain of the receptor (Fujikawa et al., 2016). However, this inhibitor did not influence MG, NIRG cells or microglia when applied after NMDA-treatment (not shown). It is likely that MDKi and SCB4380 had poor cellular permeability and these drugs failed to adequately diffuse into the retina.

We next applied an inhibitor of MDK-signaling, sodium orthovanadate (Na_3VO_4) that suppresses the activity of tyrosine phosphatases, including PTPRZ1 (Qi et al., 2001; Sakaguchi et al., 2003), which was predominantly expressed by NIRG cells, amacrine cells, and some bipolar cells (Fig. 2c). It should be noted that this drug can impact the function of tyrosine phosphatases in addition to PTPRZ1. Application of Na_3VO_4 after NMDA significantly reduced numbers of proliferating MGPCs (Fig. 3.5a,b). In addition, treatment with Na_3VO_4 significantly increased numbers of NIRG cells in the IPL (Fig. 3.5c,d) and increased numbers of dying cells (Fig. 3.5e,f). Despite this increase in retinal damage, proliferation of MGPCs was reduced in response to Na_3VO_4 after NMDA-induced damage (Fig. 3.5a,b).

We next examined the specificity of Na_3VO_4, by testing whether Na_3VO_4 blocked the effects of MDK on damaged retinas. Comparison across treatment groups (NMDA alone, NMDA + Na_3VO_4, NMDA + MDK, and NMDA + Na_3VO_4 + MDK) revealed a significant decrease in MGPCs in eyes treated with Na_3VO_4 and MDK alone (Fig. 3.5g,h). With the combination of MDK and Na_3VO_4 there was a significant increase in proliferating MGPCs relative to treatment with MDK or Na_3VO_4 alone (Fig. 3.5h). However, this level was not increased relative to levels seen with NMDA alone (Fig. 3.5h). In addition, the combination of MDK and Na_3VO_4 resulted in no significant difference in numbers of TUNEL$^+$ dying cells compared to NMDA alone (Fig 5i). These findings suggest that the effects of MDK and Na_3VO_4 upon proliferating MGPCs and numbers of dying neurons are mediated by overlapping targets.

Inhibitors of signaling though Integrin-Beta (ITGB) reduce MGPC formation in chick retina

MDK has been found to bind and signal through Integrin-Beta 1 (ITGB1) (Muramatsu et al., 2004). ITGB1 signaling occurs through different second messengers including Integrin linked kinase (*ILK*), p21 activated kinase 1 (*PAK1*), cell division factor 42 (*CDC42*), protein phosphatase 2a (PP2A, gene: *PPP2CA*), and Git/Cat-1 (*GIT1*) regulated cytoskeleton remodeling, migration, and cellular proliferation (Bagrodia and Cerione, 1999; Ivaska et al., 1999; Kawachi et al., 2001; Kim et al., 2004; Martin et al., 2016; Mulrooney et al., 2000) (see Fig. 3.11). *PAK1* has been implicated as a cell cycle regulator that is downstream of MDK and PTN signaling (Kawachi et al., 2001). PAKs are components of the mitogen activated protein kinase (MAPK) pathway and are believed to regulate small GTP-binding proteins (CDC42 and RAC) (Bagrodia and Cerione, 1999; Frisch, 2000) (see Fig. 3.11).

By probing scRNA-seq libraries we found that *PAK1* was widely expressed at relatively high levels in resting MG, and levels were significantly reduced in MG at different times after NMDA, and further reduced in MGPCs (Fig. 3.6a,b). Similarly, levels of *PPP2CA, CDC42, GIT1* and *ILK* were expressed at relatively high levels in resting MG, but were widely expressed at reduced levels in MGPCs and activated MG in damaged retinas (Fig. 3.6a,b). In addition, *PPP2CA, CDC42, GIT1* and *ILK* were expressed by different types of retinal neurons, NIRG cells and oligodendrocytes (Fig. 3.6a). We found that MG expressed *ITGB1* and other integrin isoforms, including *ITGA1, ITGA2, ITGA3* and *ITGA6* (Fig. 3.6a,b). In general, integrins were expressed at high levels in relatively few resting MG, whereas levels were reduced, but more widely expressed among activated MG, and further reduced in MGPCs (Fig. 3.6a,b). Collectively, the data demonstrates the presence of ITGB1 signaling components in MG, but the functional implications of expression changes during reprogramming are difficult to interpret.

We next tested how PAK1 and PP2A influence the formation of MGPCs in NMDA-damaged retinas. MDK-signaling is known to be modulated by the second messenger PAK1 which is upregulated in proliferating cancerous cells (Kumar et al., 2006). IPA3 is an isoform-specific allosteric inhibitor of PAK1 which prevents auto-phosphorylation (Deacon et al., 2008). Administration of IPA3 with NMDA significantly decreased numbers of proliferating MGPCs (Fig. 3.6c,d). By contrast, IPA3 had no

significant effect upon the proliferation and accumulation of NIRG cells or microglia (Fig.

3.15). Unlike Na_3VO_4, IPA3 had no impact on numbers of TUNEL[+] cells compared to

those seen in retinas treated with NMDA alone (Fig. 3.15). Since *PAK1* expression was

most prevalent in resting MG and decreased after NMDA damage, we tested whether

application of IPA3 prior to NMDA influenced glial cells and neuronal survival. We found

that IPA3 prior to NMDA resulted in a significant decrease in proliferating MGPCs (Fig.

3.6e), whereas there was no significant difference in numbers of dying cells or

proliferation of microglia and NIRG cells (Fig. 3.15). Similar to the effects of IPA3, two

different inhibitors to PP2A, fostriecin and calyculin A, significantly decreased numbers

of proliferating MGPCs in NMDA-damaged retinas (Fig. 3.6f-h). Fostriecin and calyculin

A had relatively little effect upon the accumulation, reactivity, cell death and proliferation

of NIRG cells and microglia, with the exception of a small but significant decrease in

proliferating microglia with calyculin A-treatment compared to controls (Fig. 3.15).

Collectively, these findings suggest that putative signal-transducers of MDK-signaling

promote the formation of proliferating MGPCs in damaged retinas.

Insulin and FGF2 increase MDK expression while decreasing PTN expression

In the postnatal chick retina, the formation of proliferating MGPCs can be

induced by consecutive daily injections of Fibroblast growth factor 2 (FGF2) and insulin

in the absence of neuronal damage (Fischer et al., 2002b). Eyes were treated with two

or three consecutive daily doses of FGF2 and insulin and retinas were processed to

generate scRNA-seq libraries. Cells were clustered based on their gene expression in

UMAP plots and colored by their library of origin (Fig. 3.7a,b). MG were identified based on collective expression of *VIM, GLUL* and *SLC1A3* and MGPCs were identified based on expression of *TOP2A, NESTIN, CCNB2* and *CDK1* (Fig. 3.16a,b). Resting MG from saline-treated retinas formed a cluster distinct from MG from retinas treated with two- and three-doses of FGF2+insulin based on unique patterns of gene expression (Fig. 3.7b; Fig. 3.16a,b). Additionally, MG treated with 2 versus 3 doses of insulin and FGF2 were sufficiently dissimilar to follow different trajectories of gene expression in pseudotime analysis (Fig. 3.16c,d).

Similar to patterns of expression in NMDA-damaged retinas, there was a significant increase in *MDK* with growth factor-treatment as demonstrated by patterns of expression in UMAP and violin plots, and pseudotime analyses (Fig. 3.7c-e; Fig. 3.16d-f). By comparison, levels of *PTN* were significantly decreased in MG following treatment with insulin and FGF2 (Fig. 3.7c,e; Fig. 3.16d-f). Similarly, levels of *PAK1* were decreased in activated MG and MGPCs in response to growth factor treatment (Fig. 3.7d,e; Fig. 3.16e,f). *CSPG5* was widely expressed at high levels in resting MG, and was significantly reduced in MG and MGPCs following treatment with insulin and FGF2 (Fig. 3.7d,e; Fig. 3.16e, f). *ITGB1* expression was detected in many resting MG, and decreased slightly in MG and MGPCs treated with insulin and FGF2 (Fig. 3.7d,e; Fig. 3.16e,f). In sum, treatment with FGF2 and insulin in the absence of retina damage influenced patterns of expression for MDK-related genes similar to those seen in NMDA-damaged retinas.

We next isolated MG, aggregated and normalized scRNA-seq data from saline-, NMDA-, FGF2+insulin- and NMDA/FGF2+insulin-treated retinas to directly compare levels of *MDK*, *PTN* and related factors. UMAP plots revealed distinct clustering of MG from control retinas and MG from 24hrs after NMDA-treatment, whereas MG from retinas at 48 and 72hrs after NMDA and from retinas treated with insulin and FGF2 formed a large cluster with distinct regions (Fig. 3.8a-e). UMAP and Dot plots revealed distinct patterns of expression of genes associated with resting MG, de-differentiating MG, activated MG and proliferating MGPCs (Fig. 3.8c-e). Different zones, representing MGPCs in different phases of the cell cycle were comprised of cells from different times after NMDA-treatment and FGF2+insulin-treatment (Fig. 3.8e). Expression of *MDK* was most widespread and significantly upregulated in MG in damaged retinas and MGPCs compared to MG from retinas treated with insulin and FGF2 (Fig. 3.8f). Compared to levels seen in resting MG, levels of *PTN* were reduced in activated MG from damaged retinas and MGPCs, and levels were further decreased in MG from normal and damaged retinas that were treated with insulin and FGF2 (Fig. 3.8f); similar patterns of expression were seen for *PAK1, CSPG5, ITGB1, PPP2CA* and *CDC42*. By contrast, levels of *SDC4* were highest and most widespread in MG at 24hrs after NMDA-treatment and were relatively reduced in all other groups of MG and MGPCs (Fig. 3.8f). Collectively, these findings indicate that damaged-induced changes of *MDK*, *PTN* and related factors in MG are very dramatic, and these changes in relative expression levels in MG are dampened by insulin and FGF2 whether applied to undamaged or damaged retinas.

Since growth factor treatment induces significant changes in expression of MDK-related genes, similar to that with NMDA damage, we tested whether treatment with MDK or inhibitors influenced the formation of MGPCs, or the accumulation of NIRG cells or microglia. However, we found no significant effects of MDK or IPA3 when combined with insulin and FGF2 (Fig. 3.18). By comparison, the combination of Na3VO4 with insulin and FGF2 resulted in increased accumulation of NIRG cells and some cell death, but had no influence upon the proliferating MGPCs (Fig. 3.18).

Mdk is downregulated in MG and promotes MGPC formation in damaged mouse retinas

We next sought to assess the expression of *Mdk* and related factors in normal and NMDA-damaged mouse retinas. Comparison of the different responses of glial cells across species can indicate important factors that promote or inhibit the ability of MG to reprogram into MGPCs (Hoang et al., 2020). UMAP analysis of cells from control and NMDA-damage mouse retinas revealed discrete clusters of different cell types (Fig. 3.9a). Neuronal cells from control and damaged retinas were clustered together, regardless of time after NMDA-treatment (Fig. 3.9a). By contrast, resting MG, which included MG from 48 and 72 hrs after NMDA, and activated MG from 3, 6, 12 and 24 hours after treated were spatially separated in UMAP plots (Fig. 3.9a,b). Pseudotime analysis placed resting MG (control and some MG from 48 and 72 hrs after treatment) to the left, MG from 3 and 6 hrs after treatment to the far right, and MG from 12 and 24 hrs bridging the middle (Fig. 3.17a-d). Unlike chick MG, mouse MG rapidly downregulate *Mdk* in response to damage and this downregulation is maintained through 72 hrs after treatment (Fig. 3.9c,d). Similar to MG in the chick, *Ptn* was rapidly downregulated at 3hrs, and further downregulated at 6hrs, and expressed by relatively few MG at 12-48hrs (Fig. 3.9c,d). Unlike patterns of expression in chick, levels of *Pak1* were low in resting MG, and elevated in MG only at 3hrs after NMDA-treatment (Fig. 3.9c,d). Similar to chick MG, *Cspg5* was significantly decreased in activated MG in damaged retinas (Fig. 3.9c,d). By contrast, there were significant increases in levels of *Sdc4* and *Itgb1* in MG in damaged retinas (Fig. 3.9c,d; Fig. 3.17eg). We did not detect anaplastic lymphoma kinase (*Alk*; ENSMUSG00000055471) a putative receptor for midkine and pleiotrophin (Stoica et al., 2001) in any type of cell in the mouse retina. We further analyzed the responses of MG in damaged retinas at 48hrs after NMDA ± treatment with insulin and FGF2, which is known to stimulate the proliferation of MG (Karl et al., 2008). Treatment with FGF2 and insulin in damaged retinas significantly reduced levels of *Glul*, whereas levels of *Vim* and *Gfap* were significantly increased (Fig. 3.17h-j). By comparison, levels of *Mdk* and *Sdc4* were significantly increased in MG in retinas treated with NMDA+FGF2/insulin, whereas levels of *Ptn*, *Cspg5* and *Itgb1* were unchanged (Fig. 3.17h-j).

We next investigated the activation of different cell-signaling pathways in retinal cells in response to intravitreal delivery of MDK. Similar to findings in the chick retina, we did not detect activation of NFkB, pStat3, pSmad1/5/8, pCREB, p38 MAPK or pERK1/2. Similar to findings in the chick retina, a single injection of MDK resulted in a selective and significant upregulation of cFos and pS6 in MG in the mouse retina (Fig. 3.10a-e). Other types of retinal cells did not appear to respond to MDK with upregulation of cFos or pS6. We next tested whether intraocular injections of MDK combined with NMDA-induced damage influences the proliferation of MG in the mouse retina. Consistent with previous reports (Karl et al., 2008), there were very few proliferating MG in NMDA-damaged retinas (Fig. 3.10f,h). By contrast, application of MDK with NMDA resulted in a small, but significant increase in numbers of proliferating MG (Fig. 3.10f-h). Similar to results seen in the chick retina, application of MDK prior to NMDA significantly reduced numbers of TUNEL+ cells in the INL and GCL (Fig. 3.10i-l), suggesting that MDK is potently neuroprotective to inner retinal neurons, including ganglion cells.

Discussion:

In this study, we use scRNA-seq to investigate the role of MDK and PTN in the transition of MG to MPGCs in chick and mouse retina. The patterns of gene regulation are complex and context dependent, but the dynamic regulation of mRNA is strongly correlated with changes in protein levels and function (Liu et al., 2016). Mouse and chick MG expression differed in their response to damage, and we used small molecule inhibitors of MDK and PTN to determine the functional role of these factors on MG reprogramming.

In the chick retina, MDK expression was upregulated in maturing MG during retinal development and in postnatal MG following injury or growth factor-treatment. High levels of *MDK* expression were selectively and rapidly induced in MG following damage or treatment with insulin and FGF2, with larger increases in expression seen in damaged tissues. Addition of MDK before damage was neuroprotective and resulted in decreased numbers of proliferating MGPCs. Antagonism of MDK-signaling reduced the numbers of proliferating MGPCs, stimulated the accumulation of NIRG cells, and increased the numbers of dying cells. Na_3VO_4 and PAK1 antagonism had differential effects on NIRG cells and cell death that were context dependent. In contrast to the findings in chick, we find that *Mdk* is downregulated by MG in damaged mouse retinas.

In both chick and mouse retinas, exogenous MDK selectively induces mTOR-signaling, expression of cFos in MG and protects inner retinal neurons against excitotoxic injury. However, inner retinal neurons express PTPRZ1 and MDK may directly act to protect these cells against excitotoxic injury (Fig. 3.11).

PTN signaling in the retina

PTN and MDK are in the same family of growth factors and are both dynamically expressed in the developing, damaged, and growth factor-treated retinas. Although treatment with MDK had varying effects on MG, microglia, NIRGs, and neurons, PTN administration had no detectable effects upon retinal cells. Levels of *PTN* are high in resting MG and downregulated in response to neuronal damage or treatment with insulin and FGF2. In principle, PTN acts at the same receptors as MDK, but expression of receptor isoforms may underlie the different cellular responses to MDK and PTN. PTN has preferred binding-affinity for SDC4 and ITGB3, whereas MDK has preferred binding-affinity for SDC3 and ITGB1 (Muramatsu et al., 2004; Raulo et al., 1994; Xu et al., 2014), which are expressed by bipolar cells and MG.

PTN and MDK may induce different cellular response at the same receptors. For instance, data suggests that there may be differential receptor activity between PTN and MDK on the PTPRZ receptor. Binding of PTN to PTPRZ induces oligomerization of the receptor that reduces phosphatase activity (Fukada et al., 2006). Conversely, MDK promotes embryonic neuronal survival in a PTPRZ receptor complex, which is inhibited by Na_3VO_4 (Sakaguchi et al., 2003). Although there were no detectable PTN-mediated effects upon retinal cells, PTN may serve other important biological roles in retinal homeostasis, glial phenotype/functions, or neuroprotection in other models of retinal

damage.

Receptor expression and cells responding to MDK

The effects of MDK on retinal glia has not been studied in mammals or birds. In

acutely damaged chick retina, MG are capable of forming numerous proliferating

progenitor cells (MGPCs), but few of the progeny differentiate into neurons (Fischer and

Reh, 2001; Fischer and Reh, 2002). The reprogramming of MG into MGPCs can be

induced by FGF2 and insulin in the absence of damage through MAPK signaling

(Fischer and Reh, 2002; Fischer et al., 2002a; Fischer et al., 2002b). Similarly, IGF1,

BMP, retinoic acid, sonic hedgehog, Wnt, and Jak/Stat agonists have been observed to

enhance the formation of MGPCs (Fischer et al., 2009a; Fischer et al., 2009b; Gallina et

al., 2016; Todd and Fischer, 2015; Todd et al., 2016; Todd et al., 2017; Todd et al.,

2018). Consistent across the different signaling pathways that drive the formation of

proliferating MGPCs is the upregulation of cFos and necessity for mTor-signaling in

reprogramming MG (Zelinka et al., 2016). Previous reports have provided many

examples of MDK activating cell-signaling pathways that drive proliferation (Reiff et al.,

2011; Winkler and Yao, 2014). Accordingly, we propose that MDK-mediated cell-

signaling that results in activation of cFos and mTOR contributes to the network of

pathways that drive the formation of proliferating MGPCs in the chick retinas.

Patterns of expression for receptors suggests than glial cells and inner retinal

neurons are targets of MDK and PTN. In MG the predominant receptor is *ITGB1*,

whereas NIRGs cells express *PTPRZ1*, and amacrine and bipolar cells express a combination of *PTPRZ1* and *SDC4*. The mechanism by which ITGB1 and PTPRZ influence cell cycle progression and differentiation are distinctly different. PTPRZ promotes stem cell characteristics and ligand binding inhibits phosphatase function (Fujikawa et al., 2016; Fukada et al., 2006; Kuboyama et al., 2015). Signal transduction through ITGB1 influences cytoskeleton remodeling that is associated with cell migration and proliferation (Muramatsu et al., 2004). ITGB1 can activate or inhibit secondary messengers depending on tyrosine phosphorylation (Kim et al., 2004; Mulrooney et al., 2000; Song et al., 2014). Ligand binding to ITGB1 initiates tyrosine phosphorylation of intracellular domains, and integrin linked kinases (ILKs) activate PP2A and cell cycle kinases, such as CDC42 (Ivaska et al., 1999; Ivaska et al., 2002).It has yet to be investigated how the relative changes in expression between these factors influences reprogramming and if these changes are due to positive or negative signaling feedback. The transcriptional profiles of individual retinal cell types suggest that MDK and PTN likely have autocrine and paracrine actions that are dynamically regulated in resting and damaged retinas, and in part, manifested through MG in both chick and mouse retinas.

MDK-signaling in MG

Application of MDK prior to NMDA-induced damage decreased numbers of proliferating MGPCs and decreased numbers of dying cells. Levels of retinal damage positively correlate to the proliferative response of MG (Fischer and Reh, 2001; Fischer et al., 2004). We propose that the neuroprotective effects of MDK secondarily influenced the proliferative of MGPCs. It is possible that the addition of MDK to damaged retinas did not influence MGPCs because of "ceiling effects" wherein (i) ligand/receptor interactions are saturated, (ii) the activity of secondary messengers are saturated, or (iii) the massive upregulation of MDK by MG is not directly involved in driving the formation of proliferating MGPCs.

The phosphatase inhibitor Na_3VO_4 suppressed the formation of MGPCs and increased cell death, and these effects where blocked by addition of MDK. Unfortunately, this compound likely targeted tyrosine phosphatases in addition to PTPRZ1. However, exogenous MDK reversed the inhibitory effects of Na_3VO_4 on the proliferation of MGPCs, suggesting that MDK signaling was, in part, targeted by the Na_3VO_4. We cannot exclude the possibility that some of the Na_3VO_4 mediated effects, such as increased cell death and accumulation of NIRG cells, were mediated by inhibition of phosphatases in addition to PTPRZ1. We further investigated second messengers associated with ITGB1 receptors., including PP2A and PAK1. Inhibition of Git/Cat-1/PAK1-signaling is associated with ITGB1-mediated cytoskeleton remodeling during migration and proliferation (Martin et al., 2016; Muramatsu et al., 2004). Consistent with these observations, we found that inhibition of PAK1 and PP2A effectively suppressed the formation of MGPCs in damaged retinas. Further studies are required to identify changes in phosphorylation and expression of targets that are down-stream of PP2A activity. Collectively, these findings suggest that MDK promotes the formation of proliferating MGPCs via different receptors and cell-signaling pathways in the chick retina (Fig. 3.11).

MDK and cell-signaling inhibitors did not have significant impacts upon MG and microglia in retinas treated with insulin and FGF2. Similar to NMDA-treatment, we see significant changes in expression levels of *MDK*, *PTN*, *PAK1* and *CSPG5*, suggesting that MDK-signaling is active in undamaged retinas treated with insulin and FGF2 (see Fig. 3.7). However, direct comparison of relative expression levels of *MDK* and related genes in MG across all treatment groups indicated that: (i) although *MDK* is upregulated with insulin and FGF2, levels are much less than those seen with damage, (ii) *SDC4* is modestly induced in MG by insulin and FGF2, and (iii) levels of *PAK1, CSPG5, ITGB1, PPP2CA* and *CDC4* are further downregulated by insulin and FGF2 compared to levels in MG in damaged retinas. The diminished levels of MDK-receptors and signal transducers in MG treated with insulin and FGF2, compared to levels in MG in damaged retinas, may underlie the absence of effects of exogenous MDK and inhibitors in undamaged retinas. Collectively, these findings suggest that MDK and down-stream signaling are not required for the formation of MGPCs in undamaged retinas treated with insulin+FGF2. Alternatively, the cell-signaling pathways that are activated by MDK are the same as those activated by insulin+FGF2 and there is no net gain in second messenger activation in MG by combining these factors. This may be unique because many signaling pathways that have been implicated in regulating the formation of MGPCs in the chick retina are active following both NMDA-induced damage and treatment with insulin and FGF2. These pathways include MAPK (Fischer et al., 2009a; Fischer et al., 2009b), mTOR (Zelinka et al., 2016), Notch (Ghai et al., 2010; Hayes et al., 2007), Jak/Stat (Todd et al., 2016), Wnt/b-catenin (Gallina et al., 2016), glucocorticoid (Gallina, 2015), Hedgehog (Todd and Fischer, 2015), BMP/SMAD (Todd et al., 2017), retinoic acid (Todd et al., 2018) and NFkB-signaling (Palazzo et al., 2020a).

A well-established receptor of MDK is PTPRZ (Maeda et al., 1999). PTPRZ is a cell-surface receptor that acts as a protein tyrosine phosphatase and is known to promotes proliferation (Fujikawa et al., 2016). This receptor is activated by MDK (Sakaguchi et al., 2003), but is deactivated by the binding of PTN through dimerization and tyrosine phosphorylation (Kuboyama et al., 2015). In the chick retina, the NIRG cells predominantly express *PTPRZ1* and the accumulation of these cells in response to damage was decreased with MDK-treatment and increased by treatment with phosphatase inhibitor Na_3VO_4 (Fig. 3.11). The accumulation of NIRG cells may result, in part, from migration, as MDK has been associated with migration and process elongation in different cell types (Ichihara-Tanaka et al., 2006; Kuboyama et al., 2015; Qi et al., 2001). Given that nothing is currently known about the specific functions of NIRG cells, it is difficult to infer how MDK-signaling in these glia impacts the reprogramming of MG or function/survival of retinal neurons.

MDK and reprogramming of MG into MGPCs

There has been significant investigation into the different cell-signaling pathways involved in the reprogramming of MG into proliferating MGPCs. IGF1, BMP, retinoic acid, HB-EGF, sonic hedgehog, Wnt, and CNTF are known to enhance the formation of MGPCs (Fischer et al., 2009a; Fischer et al., 2009b; Gallina et al., 2016; Todd and Fischer, 2015; Todd et al., 2016; Todd et al., 2017; Todd et al., 2018). The roles of these different pathways are similar in chick and zebrafish models of retinal regeneration, despite different capacities for neurogenesis (Goldman, 2014; Wan and

Goldman, 2016). MDK has been implicated as an important factor for reprogramming and cellular proliferation of MGPCs (Ang et al., 2020; Gramage et al., 2015; Nagashima et al., 2019a; Nagashima et al., 2019b). In the chick model, different inhibitors to PAK1, PP2A, and PTPRZ1 had relatively modest impacts on the formation of MGPCs. Although exogenous MDK likely added nothing to already saturated levels in damaged retinas, MDK or PTN alone were not sufficient to induce the formation of MGPCs in the absence of damage when levels of MDK were low. These findings suggest that MDK signaling is not a primary signaling component to drive the formation of MGPCs in chick, unlike the key role for MDK seen in zebrafish (Gramage et al., 2015; Nagashima et al., 2019b). In the chick, our findings suggest that MDK has pleiotropic roles and serves to both minimize neuronal cell death after damage and regulate the accumulation of NIRG cells. Similar to effects seen in chick MG, MDK stimulated mTor-signaling and cFos expression in mouse MG, but only induced a modest increase in numbers of proliferating MGPCs in damaged retinas. The neurogenic potential of these proliferating MG remains to be determined, but is likely to be very low given previous reports of MG-mediated regeneration in the rodent retina (Karl et al., 2008; Ooto et al., 2004).

Conclusions:

MDK and *PTN* are highly expressed by maturing MG in embryonic retinas. *MDK* is downregulated while *PTN* remains highly expressed by resting MG in the retinas of hatched chicks. Similarly, in mature mouse retinas *PTN* and *MDK* were highly expressed by mature resting MG. When MG are stimulated by growth factors or neuronal damage in chick retinas, *MDK* is robustly upregulated whereas *PTN* is downregulated. By contrast, *MDK* and *PTN* are both downregulated by MG in damaged mouse retinas. Exogenous MDK had significant effects upon proliferating glia, formation of MGPCs, and glial reactivity, whereas we did not detect cellular responses to exogenous PTN. When applied before excitotoxic injury, MDK conveyed survival-promoting effects upon inner retinal neurons in both chick and mouse models. Inhibitors of ITGB1-signaling reduced MGPC formation and phosphatase inhibitor Na_3VO_4 over-rode the effects of MDK upon neuronal survival and MGPC formation. These effects were limited to damaged retinas, whereas in undamaged retinas treated with insulin+FGF2 these effects were not observed despite dynamic changes in expression of *MDK* and related genes. Although MDK activated cFos and mTor-signaling in MG in both chick and mouse retinas, MDK had a very modest effect in stimulating the dedifferentiation and proliferation of MG in damaged mouse retinas. Overall, the upregulation of *MDK* in the chick retina is among the largest increases in gene expression detected in MG maturation or after neuronal damage, implying significant multifactorial functions in the context of development, reprogramming, and glial responses to tissue damage.

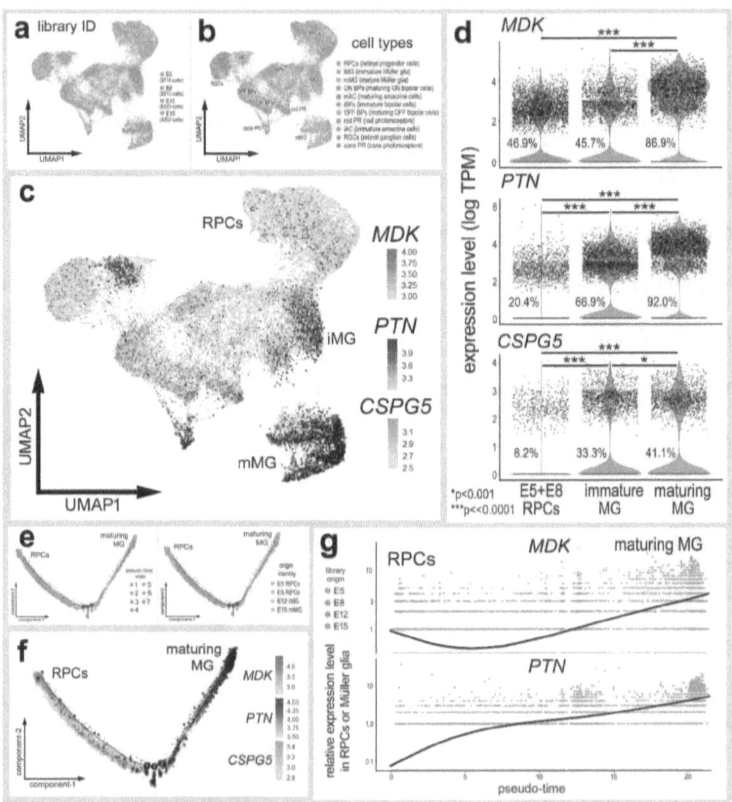

Figure 3.1. Maturing MG upregulate *MDK*, *PTN,* and *CSPG5* in embryonic chick retina. scRNA-seq was used to identify patterns of expression of *MDK*, *PTN* and putative receptor *CSPG5* among embryonic retinal cells at four stages of development (E5, E8, E12, E15). UMAP-ordered clusters of cells were identified by expression of hallmark genes (**a,b**). A heatmap of *MDK*, *PTN* and *CSPG5* illustrates expression profiles in different developing retinal cells (**c**). Each dot represents one cell and black dots indicate cells with 2 or more genes expressed. The upregulation of MDK and PTN in RPCs and maturing MG is illustrated with violin plot (**d**). The number on each violin

indicates the percentage of expressing cells. The transition from RPC to mature MG is modelled with pseudotime ordering of cells with early RPCs to the far left and maturing MG to the right of the pseudotime trajectory (**e**). *MDK* and *PTN* are upregulated in MG during maturation as illustrated by the pseudotime heatmap (**f**) and pseudotime plot (**g**). Significant difference (*p<0.01, **p<0.0001, ***p<<0.0001) was determined by using a Wilcox rank sum with Bonferroni correction. RPC – retinal progenitor cell, MG – Müller glia, iMG – immature Müller glia, mMG - mature Müller glia.

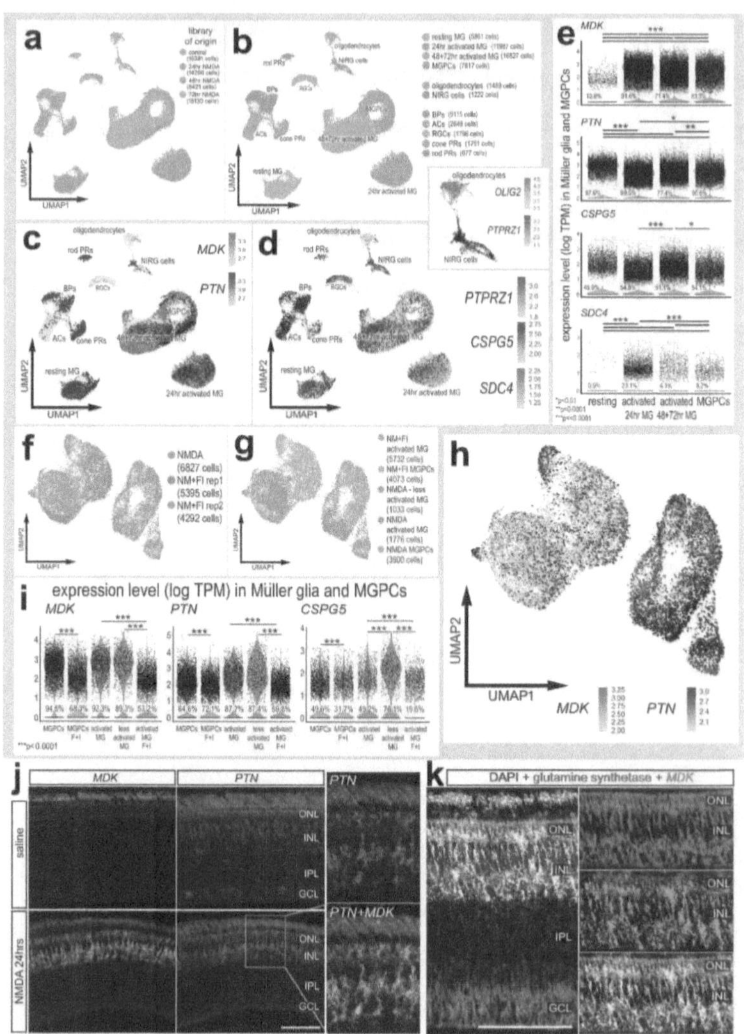

Figure 3.2. Chick MG robustly upregulate MDK and putative receptors following acute

injury. scRNA-seq was used to identify patterns of expression of MDK-related genes

among acutely dissociated retinal cells with the data presented in UMAP plots (**a-d, f, g,**

h) and violin plots (**e,i**). Control and treated scRNA-seq libraries were aggregated from 24hr, 48hr, and 72hr after NMDA-treatment (**a**). UMAP-ordered cells formed distinct clusters with MG and MGPCs forming distinct clusters (**b**). Expression heatmaps of *MDK*, *PTN*, and receptor genes *PTPRZ1*, *CSPG5*, and *SDC4* demonstrate patterns of expression in the retina, with black dots representing cells with 2 or more genes (**c,d**). In addition to NMDA, retinas were treated with insulin and FGF2 and expression levels of *MDK*, *PTN*, and *CSPG5* were assessed in MG and MGPCs (**f-i**). UMAP and violin plots illustrate relative levels of expression in MG and MGPCs treated with NMDA alone or NMDA plus insulin and FGF2 (**h,i**). Violin plots illustrate levels of gene expression and significant changes (*p<0.1, **p<0.0001, ***p<<0.0001) in levels were determined by using a Wilcox rank sum with Bonferroni correction. The number on each violin indicates the percentage of expressing cells. scRNA-seq was validated using fluorescent in-situ hybridization for *MDK* (green) and *PTN* (red) before and 24hrs after NMDA-treatment (**j**). MDK transcripts upregulated after NMDA-treatment colocalized with immunoreactivity for glutamine synthetase (**k**).

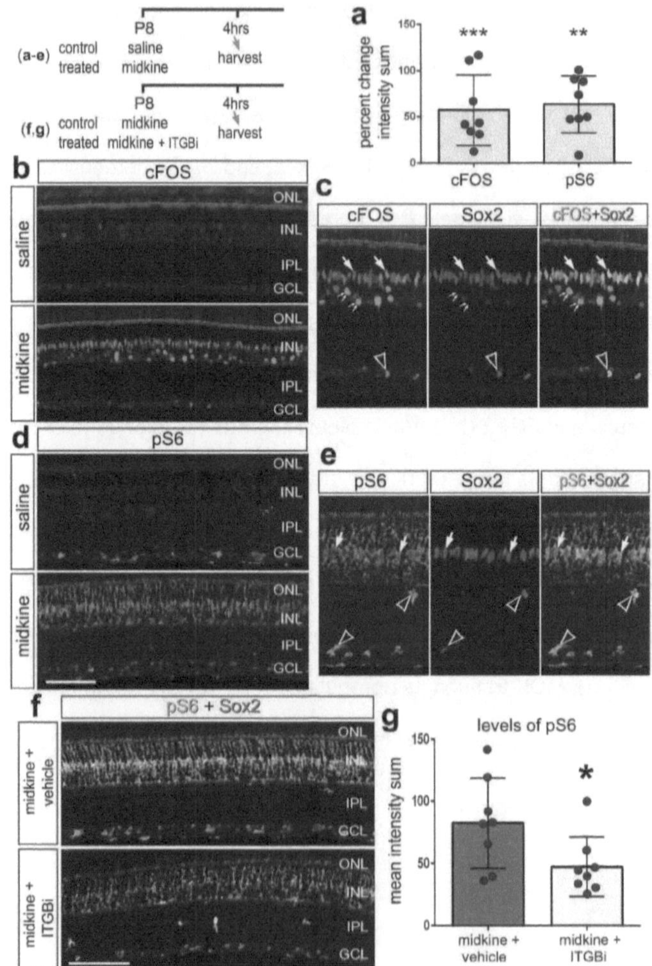

Figure 3.3. MDK activates cFos and pS6 mediated cell-signaling in chick MG. A single intraocular injection of MDK was delivered and retinas were harvested 4 hours later. The histogram in **a** represents the mean percent change (±SD) in intensity sum for cFos and pS6 immunofluorescence. Each dot represents one biological replicate retina.

Significance of difference (**p<0.01, ***p<0.001) was determined by using a paired *t*-test. Sections of saline (control) and MDK-treated retinas were labeled with antibodies to cFos (green; **b,c**), pS6 (green; **d,e**) and Sox2 (magenta; **c,e**). Arrows indicate the nuclei of MG, small double-arrows indicate the nuclei of amacrine cells, and hollow arrowheads indicate the nuclei of presumptive NIRG cells. An identical paradigm with the addition of ITGB1 signaling inhibitors fostriecin & calyculin measured changes in pS6 signaling in MG (**f**) and was quantified for intensity changes (**g**). The calibration bar (50 µm) in panel **d** applies to **b** and **d**. Abbreviations: ONL – outer nuclear layer, INL – inner nuclear layer, IPL – inner plexiform layer, GCL – ganglion cell layer.

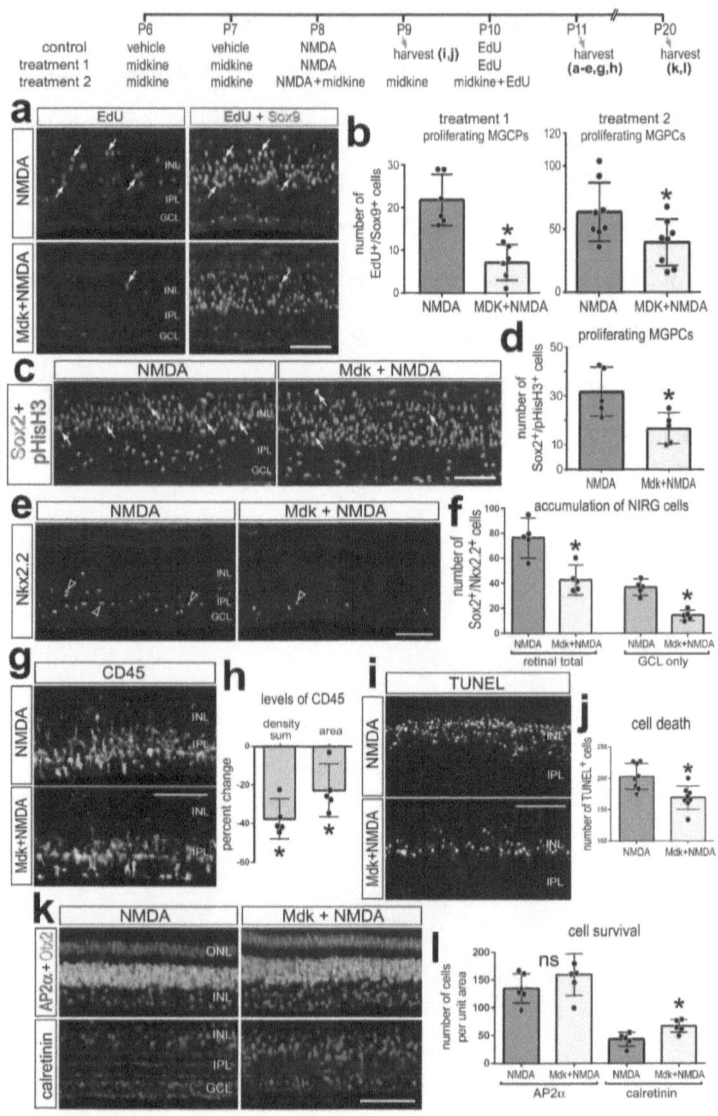

Figure 3.4. MDK treatment prior to NMDA reduces numbers of proliferating MGPCs, suppresses the accumulation of NIRG cells, and increases neuronal survival. Eyes were

injected with MDK or saline at P6 and P7, and NMDA at P8. Some retinas were harvested at P9, whereas other eyes were injected at P10 with EdU and retinas harvested 4hrs later, 24hrs later at P11 or 10 days later at P20. Sections of the retina were labeled for EdU (red) and Sox9 (green; **a**), phospho-Histone H3 (pHisH3; magenta) and Sox2 (green; **c**), Nkx2.2 (**e**), CD45 (**g**), TUNEL (**i**), and AP2α (red) and Otx2 (green) or calretinin (red; **k**). Arrows indicate nuclei of proliferating MGPCs, and hollow arrowheads indicate TUNEL-positive cells. The histogram/scatter-plots **b, d, f, j** and **l** illustrate the mean number of labeled cells (±SD). The histogram in **h** represents the mean percent change (±SD) in density sum and area for CD45 immunofluorescence. Each dot represents one biological replicate. Significance of difference (*p<0.01) was determined by using a paired *t*-test. The calibration bars panels **a, c, e, g, i** and **k** represent 50 µm. Abbreviations: ONL – outer nuclear layer, INL – inner nuclear layer, IPL – inner plexiform layer, GCL – ganglion cell layer.

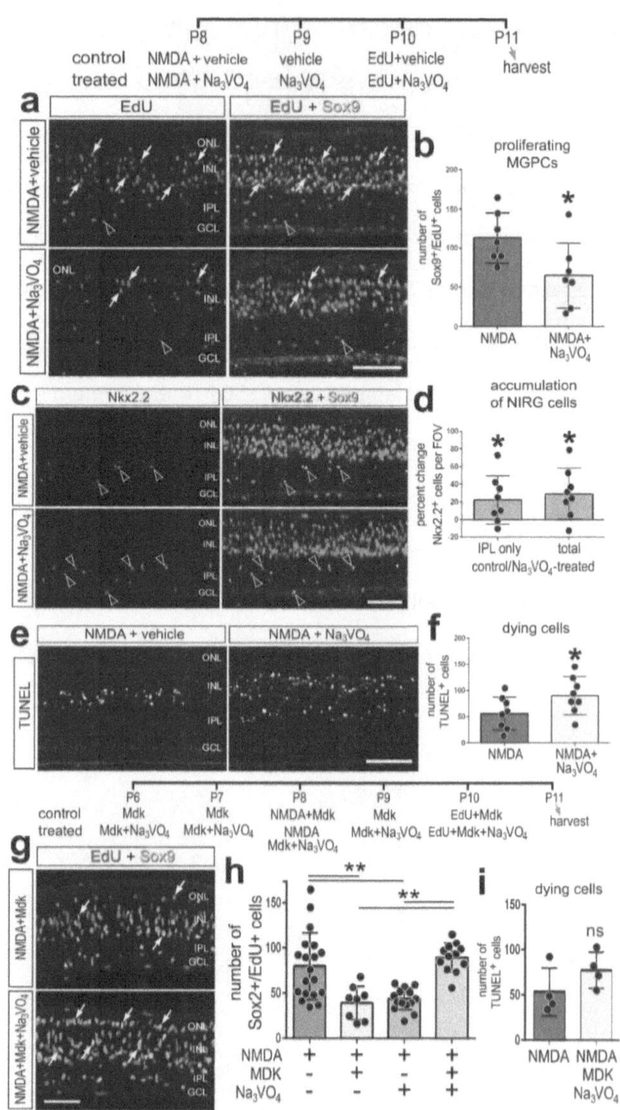

Figure 3.5. Sodium orthovanadate in NMDA-damaged retinas suppressed the formation

of MGPCs, increases numbers of dying cells, and stimulates the accumulation of NIRG cells. Eyes were injected with NMDA and Na$_3$VO$_4$ tyrosine phosphatase inhibitor or vehicle at P8, inhibitor or vehicle at P9, EdU at P10, and retinas harvested at P11. Sections of the retina were labeled for EdU (red) and Sox9 (green; **a, g**), Nkx2.2 and Sox9 (green; **c**), or TUNEL (**e**). Arrows indicate nuclei of proliferating MGPCs (**a,g**) and hollow arrowheads indicate NIRG cells (**c**). The histogram/scatterplots in **b**, **d, f, h** and **i** illustrate the mean (±SD) number of labeled cells. Each dot represents one biological replicate. Significance of difference (*p<0.05) was determined by using a paired *t*-test. The calibration bars panels **a**, **c, e** and **g** represent 50 µm. Abbreviations: ONL – outer nuclear layer, INL – inner nuclear layer, IPL – inner plexiform layer, GCL – ganglion cell layer.

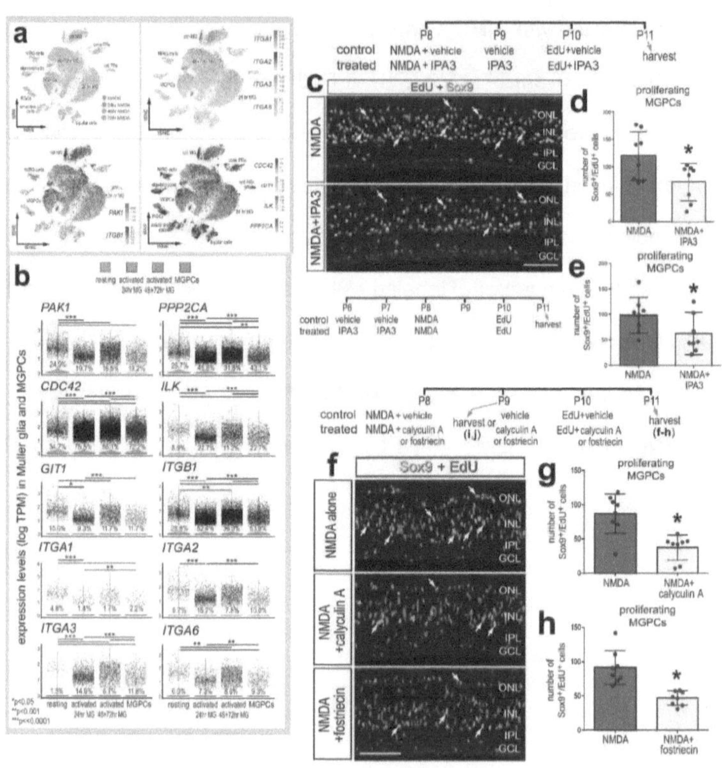

Figure 3.6. ITGB1 signaling inhibitors reduce the formation of chick MGPCs after

NMDA damage. scRNA-seq libraries (Fig. 3.2) were probed for patterns of expression

of integrin alpha/beta isoforms and associated signaling ITGB1 molecules p21

associated kinase-1 (PAK1), protein phosphatase 2a catalytic subunit alpha (PPP2CA),

integrin linked kinase (ILK), and ARF GTPase-activating protein (GIT1). tSNE plots

demonstrate patterns of expression of *PAK1, ITGB1, ITGA1, ITGA2, ITGA3, ITGA6,*

ITGAV, CAT, CDC42, GIT1, ILK and *PPP2CA* (**a**). Violin/scatter plots indicate

significant differences (*p<0.01, **p<0.001, ***p<<0.001; Wilcox rank sum with

Bonferroni correction) in expression of *PAK1, ITGB1, ITGA1, ITGA2, ITGA3, ITGA6, ITGAV, CAT, CDC42, GIT1, ILK* and *PPP2CA* among MG and MGPCs (**b**). The number on each violin indicates the percentage of expressing cells. PAK1-specific inhibitor IPA3 was injected with and following NMDA (**c**,**d**) or before NMDA (**e**) and analyzed for proliferation of MGPCs. Alternatively, PP2A-specific inhibitors calyculin A or fostriecin were injected with and following NMDA (**f-h**). Sections of the retina were labeled for EdU (red) and Sox9 (green; **c, f**). Arrows indicate nuclei of proliferating MGPCs (**a,g**). The histogram/scatterplots in **d, e, g** and **h** illustrate the mean (±SD) number of labeled cells. Each dot represents one biological replicate. Significance of difference (*p<0.05) was determined by using a paired *t*-test. Arrows indicate nuclei of proliferating MGPCs (**c,f**). The calibration bar panels **c** and **f** represent 50 µm. Abbreviations: ONL – outer nuclear layer, INL – inner nuclear layer, IPL – inner plexiform layer, GCL – ganglion cell layer, ns – not significant.

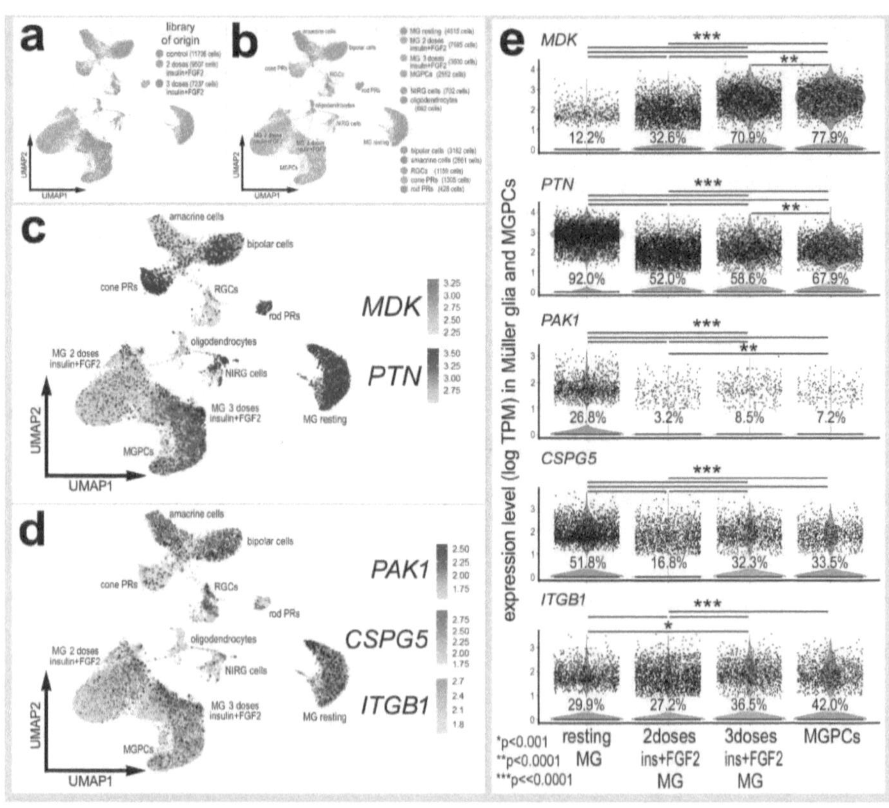

Figure 3.7. Insulin and FGF2 induce *MDK* and putative MDK-receptors in chick retinas. scRNA-seq was used to identify patterns of expression of MDK-related genes among cells in saline-treated retinas and in retinas after 2 and 3 consecutive doses of FGF2 and insulin (**a,b**). In UMAP plots, each dot represents one cell, and expressing cells indicated by colored heatmaps of gene expression for *MDK, PTN, PAK1, CSPG5* and *ITGB1* (**c,d**). Black dots indicate cells with expression of two or more genes. (**e**) Changes in gene expression among UMAP clusters of MG and MGPCs are illustrated with violin plots and significance of difference (*p<0.1, **p<0.0001, ***p<<0.0001)

determined using a Wilcox rank sum with Bonferroni correction. The number on each violin indicates the percentage of expressing cells.

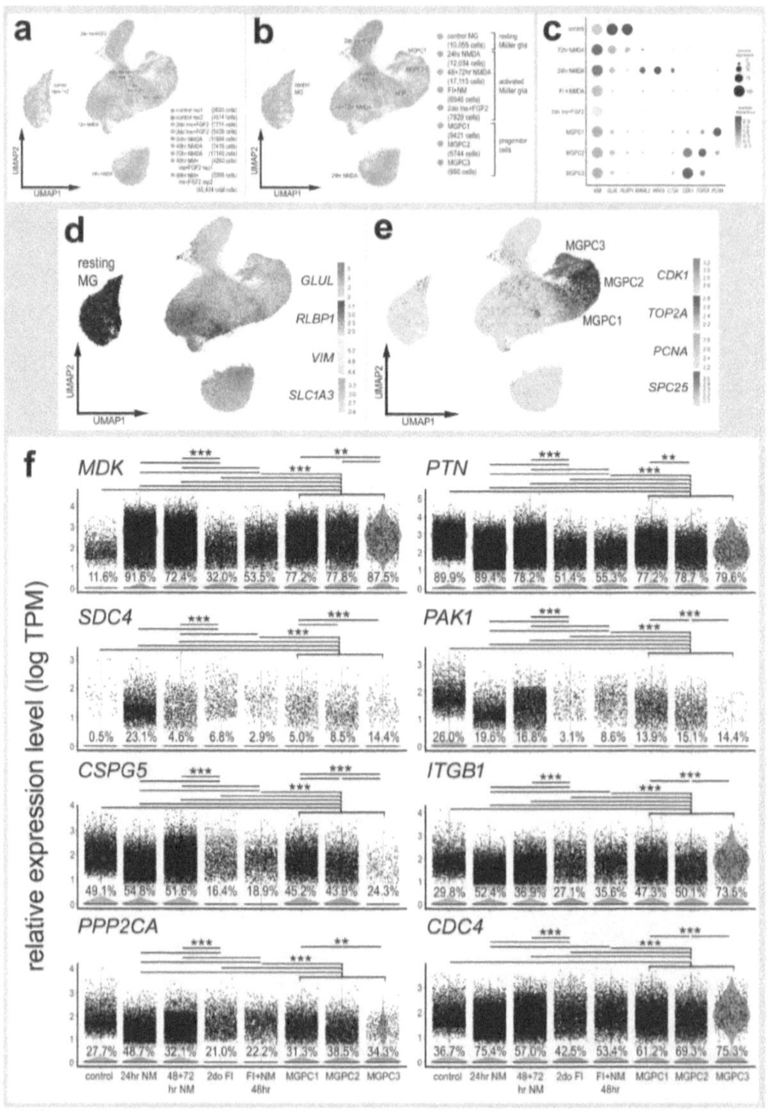

Figure 3.8. Various reprogramming treatments induce *MDK*, ITGB1, CDC4, while repressing PTN, PAK1, and CSPG5 in chick MGPCs. In UMAP and violin plots each dot

represents one cell. MG were bioinformatically isolated from 2 biological replicates for control retinas and retinas treated with 2 doses of insulin and FGF2, 3 doses of insulin and FGF2, 24 hrs after NMDA, 48 hrs after NMDA, 48hrs after NMDA + insulin and FGF2, and 72 hrs after NMDA. UMAP analysis revealed distinct clusters of MG which includes control/resting MG, activated MG from retinas 24hrs after NMDA treatment, activated MG from 2 doses of insulin and FGF2, activated MG from 3 doses of insulin FGF2 and NMDA at different times after treatment, activated MG returning toward a resting phenotype from 48 and 72 hrs after NMDA-treatment, and 3 regions of MGPCs. The dot plot in **c** illustrates some of the pattern-distinguishing genes and relative levels across the different UMAP-clustered MG and MGPCs. UMAP plots illustrate the distinct and elevated expression of *GLUL, RLBP, VIM* and *SLC1A3* in resting MG (**d**) and *CDK1, TOP2A, PCNA* and *SPC25* in different regions of MGPCs (**e**). Violin plots in **f** illustrate relative expression levels for *MDK, PTN, SDC4, PAK1, CSPG5, ITGB1, PPP2CA* and *CDC4* in UMAP-clustered MG and MGPCs. Significance of difference (**p<0.001, ***p<<0.001) was determined by using a Wilcox rank sum with Bonferroni correction. The number on each violin indicates the percentage of expressing cells.

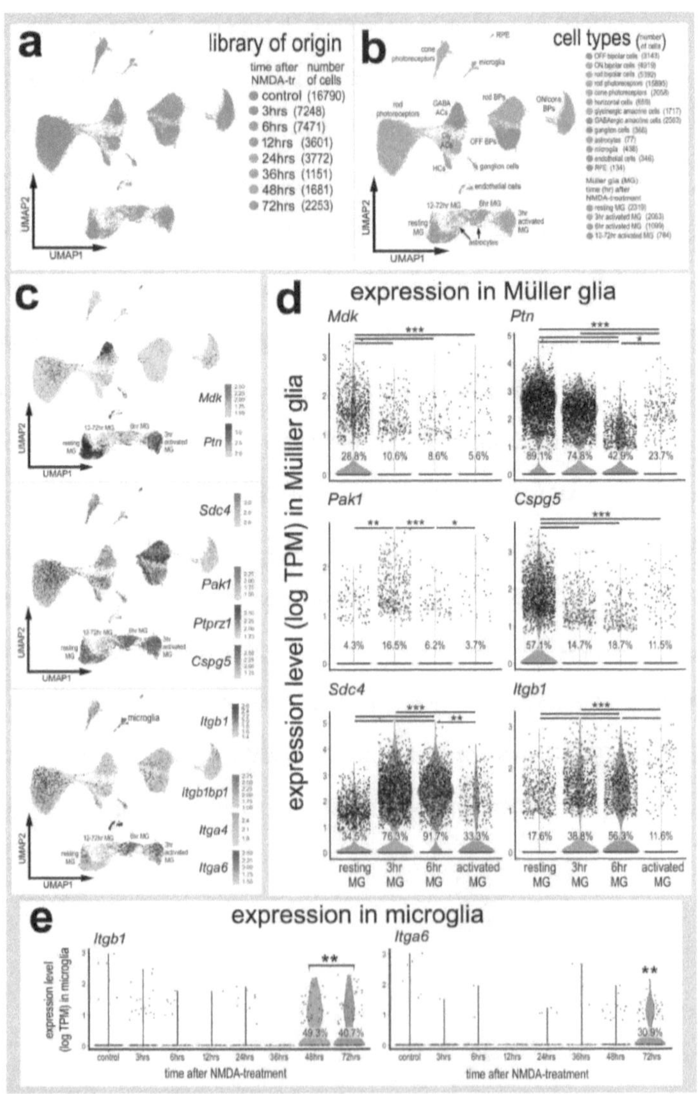

Figure 3.9. Mouse MG dynamically express *Mdk*, *Ptn* and MDK-related genes in response to NMDA damage. Cells were obtained from control retinas and from retinas

at 3, 6, 12, 24, 36, 48 and 72hrs after NMDA-treatment and clustered in UMAP plots

with each dot representing an individual cell (**a**). UMAP plots revealed distinct

clustering of different types of retinal cells; resting MG (a mix of control, 48hr and 72hr

NMDA-tr), 12-72 hr NMDA-tr MG (activated MG in violin plots), 6hrs NMDA-tr MG, 3hrs

NMDA-tr MG, microglia, astrocytes, RPE cells, endothelial cells, retinal ganglion cells,

horizontal cells (HCs), amacrine cells (ACs), bipolar cells (BPs), rod photoreceptors,

and cone photoreceptors (**b**). Cells were colored with a heatmap of expression of *Mdk,*

Ptn, Sdc4, Pak1, Ptprz1, Cspg5, Itgb1bp1, Itga4 and *Itgba6* gene expression (**c**). Black

dots indicate cells with two or more markers. In MG, changes in gene expression are

illustrated with violin/scatter plots of *Mdk, Ptn, Pak1, Cspg5, Sdc4, and Itgb1* and

quantified for significant changes (**d**) ($*p<0.01$, $**p<0.0001$, $***p<<0.001$). Similarly,

UMAP-clustered microglia were analyzed and genes *Itgb1* and *Itga6* were detected and

quantified in violin plots for cells from each library of origin (**e**). The number on each

violin indicates the percentage of expressing cells.

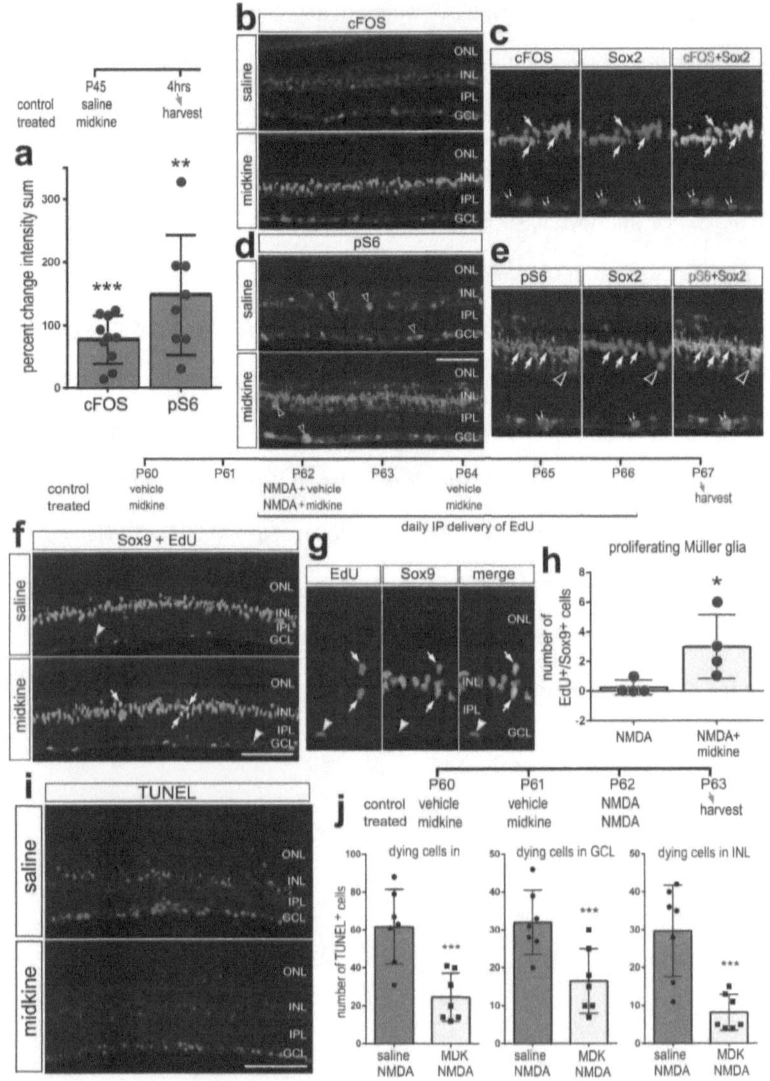

Figure 3.10. MDK activates cFos and pS6 cell-signaling in MG, stimulates proliferation

of MGPCs, and promote neuroprotection in the mouse retina. (**a-e**) A single intraocular injection of MDK was delivered and retinas were harvested 4 hours later. The histogram in **a** represents the mean percent change (±SD) in density sum and area for percentage change in intensity sum for cFos and pS6 immunofluorescence. Vertical sections of saline (control) and MDK-treated retinas were labeled with antibodies to cFos (green; **b,c**), pS6 (green; **d,e**) and Sox2 (magenta; **c,e**). (**f-h**) Treatment included intraocular injections of MDK or vehicle at P60, NMDA and MDK/vehicle at P62, MDK or vehicle at P60, EdU was applied daily by intraperitoneal (IP) injections from P62 through P66, and tissues were harvested at P67. The histogram in **h** represents the mean (±SD) number of EdU$^+$/Sox9$^+$ cells in the INL. (**i-j**) Treatment included intraocular injections of MDK or vehicle at P60 and P61, NMDA at P62, and tissues were harvested at P63. Sections of the retina were labeled for fragmented DNA using the TUNEL method (**i**). The histogram in **j** represents the mean (±SD) number of TUNEL+ cells in the retinal total, only in the GCL, or only in the INL (**j**). Each dot represents one replicate retina (**a,h,j**). Significance of difference (*p<0.05, **p<0.001, ***p<0.0001) was determined by using a paired two-way *t*-test. Arrows indicate the nuclei of MG, arrowheads indicate EdU$^+$/Sox9$^-$ cells (presumptive proliferating microglia), hollow arrowheads indicate pS6+ inner retinal neurons, and small double-arrows indicate the nuclei of Sox2+ cholinergic amacrine cells. The calibration bar (50 µm) in panel **d** applies to **b** and **d**. Abbreviations: ONL – outer nuclear layer, INL – inner nuclear layer, IPL – inner plexiform layer, GCL – ganglion cell layer.

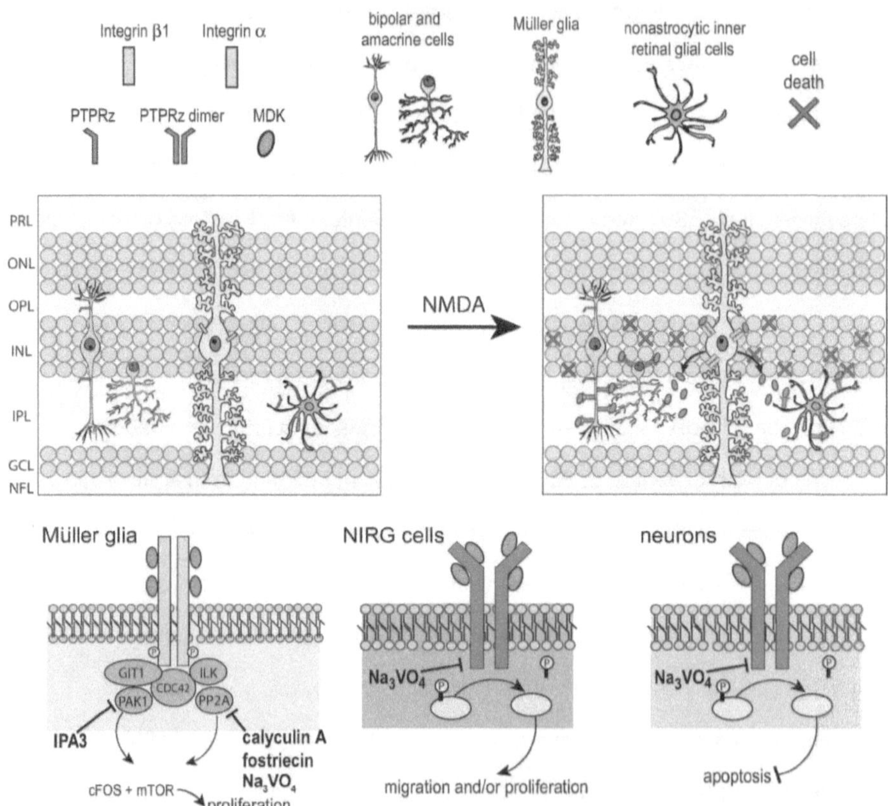

Figure 3.11. Schematic summary of MDK-signaling in normal and NMDA-damaged retinas. Patterns of expression, determined by scRNA-seq, are shown for Integrin β1, Integrin α, PTPRZ1, PAK1 and MDK in MG, NIRG cells and inner retinal neurons. Although GIT1, ILK, CDC42, and PP2A (*PPP2CA)* were widely expressed by nearly all retinal cells (according to scRNA-seq data; see Fig 6a), signaling through Integrins is shown only in MG because *ITG's* were largely confined to MG. Putative sites of action are shown for small-molecule inhibitors, including IPA3, calyculin A, fostriecin and

Na_3VO_4. Abbreviations: PRL – photoreceptor layer, ONL – outer nuclear layer, INL – inner nuclear layer, IPL – inner plexiform layer, GCL – ganglion cell layer, NFL – nerve fiber layer.

Chapter 4

Cannabinoid signaling promotes Müller glia reprogramming

Introduction

The endocannabinoid (eCB) system has been well-studied in the visual system
and is known to modulate the physiologic functions of ocular tissues, including the retina
(reviewed by (Schwitzer et al., 2016). The eCB system consists of cannabinoid
receptors 1 and 2 (*CNR1, CNR2*), endogenous ligands 2-Arachidonoylglycerol (2-AG)
and Arachidonoylethanolamide (AEA), and the enzymes that control ligand synthesis
and degradation. The eCB pathway has been identified in the retinas of different
vertebrates including embryonic chick (da Silva Sampaio et al., 2018), goldfish (Yazulla
et al., 2000), rat (Yang et al., 2016), bovine (Bisogno et al., 1999), porcine (Matsuda et
al., 1997), mouse (Hu et al., 2010), and human (Straiker et al., 1999a). The expression
of CNR1 and CNR2 receptors in the central nervous system varies across species but
typically includes distinct types of neurons, astrocytes, microglia, and Müller glia.
Activation of eCB receptors is known to modulate neurotransmission (Diana and
Bregestovski, 2005), synaptic plasticity (Xu and Chen, 2015), neuroinflammation
(Centonze et al., 2007), and neuroprotection (Slusar et al., 2013).

Müller glia (MG) are thought to play a role in regulating eCBs in the retina. Both
CNR1 and CNR2 receptors have been identified in goldfish MG (Yazulla et al., 2000),
and CNR2 receptors have been identified in the retinas of vervet monkeys (Bouskila et
al., 2013). eCBs have been shown to modify activity or suppress T-type voltage gated
calcium channels in rat MG (Yang et al., 2016) and modulate the inflammatory microenvironment (Silverman and Wong, 2018b; Todd et al., 2019). MG possess pathogen-
and damage-associated molecular pattern (PAMP/DAMP) receptors to respond to
pathological conditions (Kumar and Shamsuddin, 2012; Kumar et al., 2013;

Shamsuddin and Kumar, 2011). Activation leads to the secretion of pro-inflammatory cytokines to facilitate the migration and activation of macrophages and microglia (Inoue et al., 1996). At the same time, retinal microglia become reactive and coordinate inflammation with MG, which results in NF-kB activation, concomitant reactive gliosis, and formation of MGPCs (Palazzo et al., 2019). However, MG also produce anti-inflammatory signals such as TGF-B2 (Palazzo et al., 2020a) and TIMP3 (Campbell et al., 2019) to suppress inflammation. eCBs are believed to have anti-inflammatory actions within the central nervous system (Nagarkatti et al., 2009). Little is known about how eCBs influence inflammation in the retina and whether eCBs impact the ability of MG to reprogram into MG-derived progenitor cells (MGPCs).

The impact of inflammatory signals on MG is context specific, dependent on the combination of cytokines and the model of damage. In zebrafish, TNFα (Iribarne et al., 2019) and IL-6 (Zhao et al., 2014b) are necessary to for MG to transition from a reactive state into a proliferating progenitor cells. However, in the chick, TNF alone does not induce MGPCs and activation of the NF-kB pathway inhibits the formation of MGPCs (Palazzo et al., 2020a). In damaged mouse retinas, reactive MG rapidly transition into a gliotic state and are forced back into a resting state, in part, by regulatory networks involving NF-kB and NFI transcription factors (Hoang et al., 2020). In chick retinas, MGPCs fail to form when microglia are ablated (Fischer et al., 2014b), and the effects of NF-kB inhibition are reversed and promote the formation of MGPCs (Palazzo et al., 2020a). This suggests that there is an important balance of inflammatory cytokines and timing of signals required to drive the reprogramming of MG to dedifferentiate and proliferate as MGPCs. It is currently thought that rapid induction of microglial reactivity is required to "kick-start" MG reactivity as an initial step of reprogramming (Mumm paper; Fischer et a., 2014; Palazzo et al., 2020), whereas sustained elevated microglial reactivity suppresses the neuronal differentiation of progeny produced by MGPCs (Todd et al., 2020).

In this study we investigate the roles of eCBs in glial reactivity, inflammation and reprogramming of MG in the chick retina. Using scRNA-seq, we analyze the patterns of expression genes in the eCB system, and changes in these genes following retinal damage. Further, we apply pharmacological agents to activate or inhibit eCB-signaling and assess changes in glial phenotype and reprogramming of MG into proliferating MGPCs.

Methods and Materials:

Animals:

The animals approved in these experiments followed guidelines established by the National Institutes of Health and IACUC at The Ohio State University. P0 wildtype leghorn chicks (*Gallus gallus domesticus*) were obtained from Meyer Hatchery (Polk, Ohio). Post-hatch chicks were housed in stainless-steel brooders at 25°C with a diurnal cycle of 12 hours light, 12 hours dark (8:00 AM-8:00 PM) and provided water and Purina[tm] chick starter *ad libitum*.

Intraocular injections:

Chicks were anesthetized with 2.5% isoflurane mixed with oxygen from a non-rebreathing vaporizer. The intraocular injections were performed as previously described (Fischer et al., 1998). With all injection paradigms, both pharmacological and vehicle treatments were administered to the right and left eye respectively. Compounds were injected in 20 ml sterile saline with 0.05 mg/ml bovine serum albumin added as a carrier. Compounds included: NMDA (500nmol dose high dose, 60nmol low dose; Sigma-Aldrich), JJKK048 (0.25mg/dose Sigma-Aldrich), ARN19874 (0.25mg/dose AOBIOUS), rimonabant (0.25mg/dose Sigma-Aldrich), PF 04457845 (0.25mg/dose Sigma-Aldrich), Orlistat (0.25mg/dose Sigma-Aldrich), URB 597 (0.25mg/dose Sigma-Aldrich). 5-Ethynyl-2´-deoxyuridine (EdU) was intravitreally injected to label the nuclei of proliferating cells. Injection paradigms are included in each figure.

Enzyme-linked Immunosorbent Assay

Endocannabinoids were extracted from retinal tissue and screened for 2-AG levels using a direct competitive enzyme linked immunosorbent assay (MyBioSource). Three retinas were extracted from each treatment group and placed in 5:3 homogenization solution (formic acid pH = 3): extraction solution (9:1 ethylacetate:hexane) on ice. The tissue was homogenized with high intensity sonication on ice, frozen at -20, and the nonaqueous fraction was removed for evaporation and rehydration in DMSO. The lipid extract was applied to the wells of ELISA and the protocol was followed per the manufacturer's instructions.

Single Cell RNA sequencing of retinas

Retinas were obtained from embryonic, postnatal chick, and adult mouse retinas. Isolated retinas were dissociated in a 0.25% papain solution in Hank's balanced salt solution (HBSS), pH = 7.4, for 30 minutes, and suspensions were frequently triturated.

The dissociated cells were passed through a sterile 70µm filter to remove large
particulate debris. Dissociated cells were assessed for viability (Countess II; Invitrogen)
and cell-density diluted to 700 cell/µl. Each single cell cDNA library was prepared for a
target of 10,000 cells per sample. The cell suspension and Chromium Single Cell 3' V2
reagents (10X Genomics) were loaded onto chips to capture individual cells with
individual gel beads in emulsion (GEMs) using 10X Chromium Controller. cDNA and
library amplification for an optimal signal was 12 and 10 cycles respectively.
Sequencing was conducted on Illumina HiSeq2500 (Genomics Resource Core Facility,
John's Hopkins University) with 26 bp for Read 1 and 98 bp for Read 2. Fasta sequence
files were de-multiplexed, aligned, and annotated using the chick ENSMBL database
(GRCg6a, Ensembl release 94) and Cell Ranger software. Gene expression was
counted using unique molecular identifier bar codes, and gene-cell matrices were
constructed. Using Seurat toolkits, Uniform Manifold Approximation and Projection for
Dimension Reduction (UMAP) plots were generated from aggregates of multiple
scRNA-seq libraries (Butler et al., 2018; Satija et al., 2015). Compiled in each UMAP
plot are two biological library replicates for each experimental condition. Seurat was
used to construct violin/scatter plots. Significance of difference in violin/scatter plots was
determined using a Wilcoxon Rank Sum test with Bonferroni correction. Genes that
were used to identify different types of retinal cells included the following: (1) Müller glia:
GLUL, VIM, SCL1A3, RLBP1, (2) MGPCs: *PCNA, CDK1, TOP2A, ASCL1*, (3) microglia:
C1QA, C1QB, CCL4, CSF1R, TMEM22, (4) ganglion cells: *THY1, POU4F2, RBPMS2,
NEFL, NEFM*, (5) amacrine cells: *GAD67, CALB2, TFAP2A*, (6) horizontal cells:
PROX1, CALB2, NTRK1, (7) bipolar cells: *VSX1, OTX2, GRIK1, GABRA1*, and (7) cone

photoreceptors: *CALB1, GNAT2, OPN1LW*, and (8) rod photoreceptors: *RHO, NR2E3, ARR3*. The MG have an over-abundant representation in the scRNA-seq databases. This likely resulted from capture-bias and/or tolerance of the MG to the dissociation process. scRNA-seq libraries can be queried at:

Fixation, sectioning, and immunocytochemistry:

Ocular tissues were fixed, sectioned, and labeled via immunohistochemistry as described previously (Fischer et al., 2008; Fischer et al., 2009b). Dilutions and commercial sources of antibodies used in this study are listed in table 2. Observed labeling was not due to off-target labeling of secondary antibodies or tissue autofluorescence because sections incubated with only secondary antibodies were devoid of fluorescence. Secondary antibodies included donkey-anti-goat-Alexa488/568, goat-anti-rabbit-Alexa488/568/647, goat-anti-mouse-Alexa488/568/647, goat-anti-rat-Alexa488 (Life Technologies) diluted to 1:1000 in PBS and 0.2% Triton X-100.

Labeling for EdU:

For the detection of nuclei that incorporated EdU, immunolabeled sections were fixed in 4% formaldehyde in 0.1M PBS pH 7.4 for 5 minutes at room temperature. Samples were washed for 5 minutes with PBS, permeabilized with 0.5% Triton X-100 in PBS for 1 minute at room temperature and washed twice for 5 minutes in PBS. Sections were incubated for 30 minutes at room temperature in a buffer consisting of 100 mM Tris, 8 mM $CuSO_4$, and 100 mM ascorbic acid in dH_2O. The Alexa Fluor 568 Azide (Thermo Fisher Scientific) was added to the buffer at a 1:100 dilution.

Terminal deoxynucleotidyl transferase dUTP nick end labeling (TUNEL):

The TUNEL assay was implemented to identify dying cells by imaging fluorescent labeling of double stranded DNA breaks in nuclei. The *In-Situ* Cell Death Kit (TMR red; Roche Applied Science) was applied to fixed retinal sections as per the manufacturer's instructions.

Photography, measurements, cell counts and statistics:

Microscopy images of retinal sections were captured with the Leica DM5000B microscope with epifluorescence and the Leica DC500 digital camera. High resolution confocal images were obtained with a Leica SP8 available in The Department of Neuroscience Imaging Facility at The Ohio State University. Representative images are modified to have enhanced color, brightness, and contrast for improved clarity using Adobe Photoshop. In EdU proliferation assays, a fixed region of retina was counted and average numbers of Sox2 and EdU co-labeled cells. The retinal region selected for investigation was standardized between treatment and control groups to reduce variability and improve reproducibility.

Similar to previous reports (Fischer et al., 2009a; Fischer et al., 2009b; Ghai et al., 2009), immunofluorescence was quantified by using Image J (NIH). Identical illumination, microscope, and camera settings were used to obtain images for quantification. Retinal areas were sampled from 5.4 MP digital images. These areas were randomly sampled over the inner nuclear layer (INL) where the nuclei of the bipolar and amacrine neurons were observed. Measurements of immunofluorescence were performed using ImagePro 6.2 as described previously (Ghai et al., 2009; Stanke et al., 2010; Todd and Fischer, 2015). The density sum was calculated as the total of pixel values for all pixels within thresholded regions. The mean density sum was calculated for the pixels within threshold regions from ≥5 retinas for each experimental condition. GraphPad Prism 6 was used for statistical analyses.

Measurements of immunofluorescence of CD45 in the nuclei of microglia were made by from single optical confocal sections by selecting the total area of pixel values above threshold (≥70) for CD45 immunofluorescence. Measurements were made for regions containing pixels with intensity values of 70 or greater (0 = black and 255 = saturated). The total area was calculated for regions with pixel intensities above threshold. The intensity sum was calculated as the total of pixel values for all pixels within threshold regions. The mean intensity sum was calculated for the pixels within threshold regions from ≥5 retinas for each experimental condition.

For statistical evaluation of differences across treatments, a two-tailed paired *t*-test was applied for intra-individual variability where each biological sample also served as its own control. For two treatment groups comparing inter-individual variability, a two-tailed unpaired *t*-test was applied. For multivariate analysis, an ANOVA with the associated Tukey Test was used to evaluate any significant differences between multiple groups.

Results:

Muller glia express genes related to the endocannabinoid pathway

scRNA-seq libraries were aggregated from control retinas and retinas treated with NMDA-damage and/or FGF and insulin at different times (24, 48 and 72 hrs) after treatment. These libraries were clustered and analyzed (Fig 4.8), or MG isolated and reaggregated for broad analysis of eCB genes under reprogramming conditions (Fig. 4.1a). UMAP plots of MG were generated and clusters were identified by expression of cell-distinguishing markers (Fig. 4.1a,b). Microglia were not included in these data sets because of limited sensitivity and quality control filtering. Resting MG occupied a discrete cluster of cells and expressed high levels of *GLUL, VIM, RLBP1* and *SLC1A3* (Fig. 4.1c). After damage, MG down-regulate these genes during transition to a reactive phenotype and into progenitor-like cells that up-regulate proliferation-related genes (Fig. 4.1d).

The expression of eCB-related genes in MG has been previously reported in developing chick retina (da Silva Sampaio et al., 2018). The eCB system involves receptors *CNR1* and *CNR2* and enzymes involved in the synthesis (*NAPEPLD, DAGLA* and *DAGLB*) of 2-AG and AEA from membrane phospholipids and degradation (*FAAH* and *MGLL*) of ligands to regulate levels (Fig. 4.1e). We detected *CNR1, MGLL, DAGLA, DAGLB, NAPELPD and FAAH* in MG (Fig. 4.1e,f). *CNR2* was not detected. *CNR1* was also detected at high levels in many amacrine cells and a few ganglion cells (Fig. 4.1e). *MGLL* and *NAPEPLD* were detected at high levels in many oligodendrocytes and bipolar cells, and in relatively few photoreceptors and ganglion cells (Fig. 4.1e). *CNR1* and eCB-related genes, except *FAAH*, were uniformly down-regulated in MG at 24hrs after treatment (Fig. 4.1e,f). Prevalence and levels of expression of *CNR1, MGLL* and *NAPEPLD* were increased in MG but decreased in MGPCs from retinas at 48 and 72hrs after NMDA-treatment (Fig. 4.1f).

To assess whether eCB-related genes where differentially expressed because of neuronal damage, we probed for changes in levels of expression in MG and MGPCs in retinas treated with insulin and FGF2, in the absence of damage (Fischer et al., 2009a; Fischer et al., 2009b). We generated aggregate scRNA-seq libraries from control retinas or retinas treated with 2 or 3 doses of insulin and FGF2 (Fig. 4.1g). Microglia were not included in these data sets because of limited sensitivity and quality control filtering. Similar to the distribution of MG in UMAP plots of NMDA-treated cells, MG formed distinct clusters according to growth factor treatment, and down-regulated genes characteristic of resting MG and up-regulated genes characteristic of proliferating progenitors (Fig. 4.1g-j). Although levels *CNR1* and *FAAH* in MG were not significantly changed by growth factor treatment, levels of *MGLL*, *DAGLA*, *DAGLB* and *NAPEPLD* were downregulated in MG and MGPCs by insulin and FGF2 (Fig. 4.1k,l). Collectively, these findings suggest that the expression of most eCB-related genes by MG are changed predominantly in response to neuronal damage, whereas levels of *MGLL* were prominently down-regulated by treatment with NMDA (neuronal damage) or insulin and FGF2 (no neuronal damage).

Intravitreal eCBs promote the formation of MGPCs after damage

Although patterns of gene expression can be complex and context dependent, dynamic changes in mRNA levels are strongly correlated with changes in protein levels and function (Liu et al., 2016). The ligand binding affinity of chick CNR receptors remains uncertain. Accordingly, 2-AG and AEA were co-injected into maximize the potential activation of CNR1 receptors in the retina. We tested whether co-injection of 2-

AG and AEA influenced the formation of proliferating MGPCs in damaged retinas.

Compared to numbers of proliferating MGPCs in NMDA-damaged retinas, treatment

with NMDA and eCBs resulted in a significant increase in numbers of Sox2/EdU-

positive MGPCs (Fig. 4.2a-c). Consistent with these findings, numbers of proliferating

MGPCs that expressed neurofilament and phospho-histone H3 (pHH3) were

significantly increased by treatment with 2-AG and AEA (Fig. 4.2d,e). Levels of retinal

damage influence the reprogramming of MG; there is a positive correlation between

numbers of dying cells and numbers of proliferating MGPCs (Fischer and Reh, 2001;

Fischer et al., 2004). The number of TUNEL-positive cells was unchanged by 2-AG and

AEA, suggesting that levels of cell death in NMDA-damaged retinas was unaffected by

addition of eCBs (Fig4.2. f,g).

Targeting the eCB pathway influenced MG reprogramming

Since expression levels of genes associated with eCB signaling and metabolism

were changed in NMDA-damaged retinas, we investigated whether levels of eCBs were

influenced by damage or drugs that interfere with synthesis or degradation. We applied

Orlistat, an inhibitor of DAGL, to reduce eCB synthesis and JJKK-048, an inhibitor to

MGLL, to suppress eCB degradation (Hillard, 2015). By using competitive inhibition

ELISAs, we measured levels 2-AG and AEA in retinas treated with NMDA and

inhibitors. We detected low levels of 2-AG in the retina, that did not significantly change

with NMDA damage at 72 hours (Fig. 4.3a). Although we failed to detect a significant

change in 2-AG with Orlistat treatment, injections of JJKK-048 resulted in a significant

increase in retinal levels of 2-AG (Fig. 4.3a). AEA was not detectable within the

threshold range of the ELISA kit, and, thus, inhibitor treatments had no detectable impact on levels of AEA (Fig. 4.3b). Since levels of AEA fell below levels of detection we did not probe for changes in AEA-levels following treatment with inhibitors of NAPEPLD or FAAH.

We next tested whether inhibition of enzymes that produce or degrade eCBs influence glial reactivity, cell death and the formation of MGPCs (Fig. 4.3a). We also targeted the CNR1 receptor with a small molecule agonist and antagonist to further investigate whether CNR1 influences retinal cells in damaged retinas. Win-55, 212-2 (Win55) is a potent CNR agonist in humans, mice and chickens (Stincic and Hyson, 2011). Rimonabant is a potent and selective antagonist that inhibits CNR1-mediated cell-signaling (Ádám et al., 2008). (Hillard, 2015) Activation of CNR1 with Win55 increased numbers of proliferating MGPCs, whereas inhibition of CNR1 with rimonabant had the opposite effect (Fig. 4.3c,d,e). MGLL inhibitor (JJKK048), which increased levels of 2-AG (Fig. 4.3a), increased numbers of proliferating of MGPCs (Fig. 4.3f). By comparison, the DAGL inhibitor Orlistat significantly decreased numbers of MGPCs (Fig 4.3g). Overall, treatments expected to increase levels/signaling of eCBs increased MG reprogramming and treatments to decrease levels/signaling of eCBs decreased MG reprogramming.

We next targeted enzymes that influence the synthesis (NAPEPLD) or degradation (FAAH) of AEA. Inhibition of NAPELPD with ARN19784 had no effect upon numbers of proliferating MGPCs (Fig. 4.3a,b), whereas numbers of proliferating microglia were increased (Fig 4.3c,d) and numbers of proliferating NIRG cells and dying cells were decreased (Fig. 4.3e-h). By comparison, inhibition of FAAH with URB597 or PF-044 had no significant effect upon the proliferating of MGPCs, microglia and NIRG cells, or cell death (Fig. 4.3d,f,h). We bioinformatically isolated microglia from preparations using updated reagents with improved sensitivity. A fine-grain bioinformatic analysis of microglia revealed discrete clustering of resting and activated microglia (Fig. 4.3i-l), and scattered expression of *MGLL* and *NAPEPLD*, but no expression of *CNR1* (Fig. 4.5m) or *FAAH* (not shown). These data suggest that cells in chick retina support a production of 2-AG over AEA, especially in the context of damage and reprogramming. Further the reactivity of some microglia and NIRG cells, but not MG, is influenced by inhibition of NAPEPLD.

Microglia Reactivity is unaffected by changes in eCBs

Retinas have resident microglia that serve homeostatic functions and mediate inflammation in response to damage and pathogens (Silverman and Wong, 2018b). In response to excitotoxic damage in the chick, the microglia become reactive, leading to accumulation of monocytes, proliferation, and upregulation of inflammatory cytokines (Fischer et al., 2014b). Given the known association of microglia, inflammation and eCB signaling (Stella, 2009) and the dependence of MGPC formation on signals provided by reactive microglial (Fischer et al., 2014b; Palazzo et al., 2020a), we investigated the impact of drugs targeting CNR1 and 2-AG metabolism on microglia reactivity, proliferation and reactivity.

Microglia are sparsely distributed and highly ramified when quiescent, but become reactive and transiently accumulate after NMDA-treatment (Fischer et al., 2014b). We applied established metrics of microglia reactivity in the chick model (Gallina, 2015), including microglia infiltration/accumulation, proliferation, CD45-

intensity, cell area, and ramification were compared in different eCB targeted treatments. eCBs and small molecule inhibitors had no significant effect on the reactivity of microglia in damaged retinas (Fig. 4.5). Both the small molecule drugs and 2-AG/AEA did not change total numbers of CD45$^+$ cells compared to damage alone (Fig. 4.5a-c). Similarly, the number of proliferating CD45$^+$ immune cells were unaffected by eCB treatments in the damaged retina (Fig. 4.5a-c). Similarly, the area and intensity of CD45$^+$ immunolabeling were unaffected by drugs targeting eCBs (Fig. 4.5c). The individual microglia were also unchanged in their morphology (Fig. 4.5d). Using a Sholl analysis to quantify microglia shape, we quantified the maximum intersections (ramification index), mean intersections (centroid value), and maximum intersection radius (processes distribution). In damaged retinas the reactive morphology of microglia was unchanged by drugs targeting eCBs (Fig. 4.5).

The lack of effects of eCB-activation/inhibition upon microglia prompted us to probe scRNA-seq libraries that were generated with 10x genomics V3 reagents and at timepoints shortly after NMDA-treatment, when microglia are known to rapidly change expression profiles in mouse retinas (Todd et al., 2019). Resting microglia formed a distinct UMAP cluster (Fig. 4.5f). Activated microglia from 3 and 12 hrs after NMDA formed a cluster with up-regulation of TNFSF15, PPARG and IL1R2, whereas activated microglia from later times after NMDA formed discrete UMAP clusters with elevated levels of *DBI* and *AIF1L* (Fig. 4.5f). Although microglia had scattered expression of *NAPEPLD* and *MGLL*, we failed to detect significant *CNR1* expression among microglia from different treatment groups (Fig. 4.5g).

NF-kB activation is reduced in mouse MG when promoting eCB signaling

NF-kB is a transcription factor known to be a primary transductor of the innate and adaptive immunity and central mediator of the inflammatory response to pathogens and tissue damage (Liu et al., 2017). In the chick model of reprogramming, targeting the regulators of the NF-kB pathway has a significant impact on the capacity of MG to become progenitor like (Palazzo et al., 2020a). With microglia present, increasing NF-kB signaling using small molecule inhibitors reduced the formation of MGPCs.

For a readout of NF-kB signaling, we utilized the cis-NF-kB[eGFP] reporter mouse line to visualize cells where p65 is driving transcription in the nucleus (Magness et al., 2004). In undamaged retinas, NFkB reporter was observed in a few endothelial cells whereas eGFP reporter was not detected in any retinal neurons or glia (Fig. 4.6a). At 48hrs after NMDA damage significant numbers of MG express NFkB-eGFP (Fig 4.6b). Treatment with CNR1 agonist win55 or eCBs (2-AG/AEA) resulted in a significant reduction in numbers of MG that were positive for eGFP (Fig. 4.6g,h,i). To determine if changes in cell death were influenced eCBs, we performed TUNEL staining to determine that there was no change in cell death in total, or in the GCL or INL layers (Fig. 4.6f). This evidence suggests that eCBs can influence NF-kB signaling in MG, which may play a role in their capacity to reprogram into progenitor-like cells.

Discussion:

In this study we investigated the roles of eCB-signaling in the chick model of MG reprogramming. MG expressed both the CNR1 receptor and genes involved in the synthesis and degradation of eCBs. The levels of expression and proportion of MG that express these genes significantly change following damage and during the transition of

MG to a proliferating progenitor-like cell. These changes in expression imply functions for eCBs in damaged retinas and during the formation of MGPCs. Indeed, we found that reprogramming of MG into proliferating MGPCs was promoted by eCBs and by CNR1 agonists or enzyme inhibitors that increase retinal levels of 2-AG. Microglial reactivity was largely unaffected by drugs targeting eCBs and maintain a reactive phenotype in damaged retinas regardless of treatment with drugs. These findings support recent reports that the inflammatory state of MG is important to the transition from resting to reactive, and then to a progenitor-like cell (Fischer et al., 2014b; Hoang et al., 2020; White et al., 2017).

eCB signaling gene expression

In the chick retina the expression of CNR1 and MGLL has been reported in MG (da Silva Sampaio et al., 2018). In addition to expression in MG, we detected *CNR1* in MG and in a population of amacrine cells (Fig 4.8), and MGLL was detected in MG and some types of ganglion cells and oligodendrocytes. The eCB-related genes were present in MG but at low levels and only in a small proportion of MG. This pattern of expression is in contrast with the high-expressing glial markers, such as glutamine synthetase (*GLUL*), retinaldehyde binding protein 1 (*RLBP1*) and carbonic anhydrase 2 (*CA2*) that are present in all MG. We believe this may be due to sensitivity limitations of the 10X Genomics V2 reagents, that have recently been replaced with optimized V3 regents with improved transcript capture efficacy and sensitivity to detect low-copy transcripts. It is also possible that a sub-population of MG express eCB-related genes, suggesting heterogeneity among MG types. However, the eCB-expressing MG subsets are scattered homogenously in these clusters and do not correlate with unique markers indicating a biologically unique subcluster.

Elevated eCBs promote MG reprogramming

Although the roles of eCBs have been investigated in vision, little is known about how eCBs influence MG reprogramming in models of retinal regeneration. We observed that exogenous eCB increased the proportion of MG that formed proliferating MGPCs. This effect was reproduced with inhibition of MGLL with JJKK048 which degrades 2-AG into glycerol and arachidonic acid. This drug was validated to target MGLL and decrease levels of 2-AG levels in mice (Hillard, 2015), consistent with our findings that JJKK048 increased retinal levels of 2-AG. Orlistat has shown to inhibit DAGL in 2-AG synthesis humans (Bisogno et al., 2006). Although we observed a decrease in number of proliferating MGPCs with Orlistat treatment, we did not observe a significant decrease in 2-AG via ELISA. This may have resulted from the low sensitivity threshold for detecting 2-AG in the assay. These lipids represent a very small fraction of total lipids from whole-retina extracts. Alternatively, Orlistat could be targeting FASN, disrupting lipid metabolism more broadly to influence retinal levels of 2-AG (Kridel et al., 2004).

We examined whether CNR1 may have mediated eCB effects applying selective small molecule agonists and antagonists, drugs with validated specificity in the chick CNS (Ádám et al., 2008; Stincic and Hyson, 2011). We observed complimentary effects with Win55 (CNR1 agonist) increasing and rimonabant (CNR1 antagonist) decreasing numbers of proliferating MGPCs. Nevertheless, we cannot exclude the possibility that these effects are due to indirect actions at MG. For example, amacrine or ganglion cells that express CNR1 could have mediated effects on MG through secondary factors. We failed to detect CNR1 expression among microglia, NIRG cells or oligodendrocytes at timepoints shortly after NMDA-treatment.

The data support the hypothesis that MG are receptive and responsive to eCBs. In other animal models and cell types, changes in cell physiology are mediated via interactions and cross talk with other pathways, such as Notch1 (Frampton et al., 2010), mTor (Palazuelos et al., 2012), MAPK/PI-3K (Dalton et al., 2009), and Wnt signaling (Nalli et al., 2019). These cell signaling pathways are known to be active and promote the reprogramming of MG into MGPCs in the chick model (Fischer et al., 2002b; Gallina et al., 2016; Ghai et al., 2010; Zelinka et al., 2016). However, we have yet to identify the crosstalk interactions between eCB signaling and other pro-reprogramming signaling pathways. These connections may be difficult to identify in undamaged retinas given that homeostatic enzymes reduce eCBs in the microenvironment and because MG sensitivity to eCBs increases after damage by upregulating of *CNR1*.

eCBs are not neuroprotective to excitotoxic NMDA damage

eCBs have been shown to provide neuroprotection in degenerative retinal diseases (Rapino et al., 2018). Recent articles have even suggested that 2-AG can mediate neuroprotection against AMPA toxicity in the rat retina (Kokona et al., 2021). We investigated eCB-related neuroprotection because levels of retinal damage and cell death are known to influence the reprogramming of MG in to MGPCs. Although, injections of 2-AG and AEA did not impact numbers of dying cells, the CNR1 agonist

Win55 increased cell death in the chick (Fig 4.9a,b). This could result from interactions with ion channels that are known to occur with these lipid molecules (Pertwee, 2010). Alternatively, differences could be due to NMDA vs AMPA receptors. Kokona et al. (2021) reported cell death of photoreceptors with AMPA-selective agonists, which does not occur in NMDA. In other disease models where 2-AG provides neuroprotection the mode of cellular damage is slow and progressive (Centonze et al., 2007), unlike our model of NMDA-induced excitotoxicity which acute and severe.

Microglia reactivity is not influenced by eCBs

eCBs are believed to be potent anti-inflammatory drugs in the CNS (Ullrich et al., 2007). This is frequently suggested as mechanism of clinical benefit in pathological states. In the chick model of reprogramming, we have used dexamethasone GCR receptor agonist to repress the reactivity of microglia (Gallina, 2015). Similarly, treating damaged retinas with NF-kB inhibitor sulfasalazine also resulted in a decrease in the reactive proliferation of CD45[+] cells (Palazzo et al., 2020a). With eCBs and small molecule drugs, there was no evidence that the reactivity of immune cells was influenced with the exception of the NAPEPLD inhibitor. These findings are consistent with our findings that activated microglia express NAPEPLD. Retinal studies where microglial reactivity is reduced may secondarily result in neuroprotective effects since exacerbated microglial reactivity can be detrimental to neuronal survival (Fischer et al., 2015; Todd et al., 2019)

Our findings are consistent with the notion that eCB-signaling is primarily controlled and manifested through MG. However, we cannot exclude the possibility of eCB-mediated changes in production pro-inflammatory cytokines from reactive microglia in damaged retinas. The relationship between these inflammatory factors and MGPC formation is complex and time dependent. For example, decreased retinal inflammation from inhibition of microglial reactivity with glucocorticoid agonists reduced MGPC formation, whereas decreased retinal inflammation from inhibition of NFkB signaling increased MGPC formation (Gallina, 2015; Palazzo et al., 2020a). However, the impact of NFkB-signaling on the formation of MGPCs was reversed when the microglia were selectively ablated (Palazzo et al., 2020a). Pro-inflammatory factors likely directly influence MG, with evidence that MG activate NF-kB-signaling and express cytokine receptors in damaged retinas (Palazzo et al., 2020a). Further studies are required to determine the impact of pro-inflammatory signals on microglia and MG in eCB-treated retinas to better characterize the coordination between these glial cells.

eCBs repress NF-kB in mouse MG

While reporter lines for MG do not exist in the chick model, the mouse model of retinal damage was applied to the cis-NF-kB^{eGFP} mice to observe cells where p65 translocate into the nucleus and actively binds to the DNA to drive the expression of the eGFP reporter. MG are the primary cell type activating NF-kB in the damaged retina. This supports prior findings in chick that MG secrete proinflammatory cytokines such as TNF associated with NF-kB signaling (Palazzo et al., 2020a). After damage eCBs reduced the density of GFP$^+$ MG, demonstrating that through a direct or indirect mechanism eCB limit the activation of NF-kB in damaged tissue. NF-kB has been suggested to be an important signaling pathway in mouse retina that may mediate a cellular switch between reactive gliosis and de-differentiation into MGPCs (Hoang et al., 2020).

Recent studies into MG reprogramming have highlighted the importance of the interaction between microglia and MG in mouse. Hoang et al. (2020) showed how NF-kB genes serve as a distinguishing factor in mice that may upregulate reactive glial genes, or enable MG to re-enter the cell cycle and de-differentiate to improve the potential for pro-neural reprogramming. The ablation of microglia with CSF1R inhibitors had a dramatic impact on the neurogenic capacity of MG overexpressing Ascl1 (Todd et al., 2020). The absence of microglia altered the MG transcriptome to repress gliotic reactive genes. How the context, timing, and extent of immune interactions can be controlled to maximize the reprogramming capacity in mice has yet to be explored.

Conclusions:

In this study we investigated the impact of eCBs on retinal inflammation and MG reprogramming in the chick model. We found transcriptomic evidence of eCB genes expressed by MG and the expression of these genes was dynamic following injury and during the transition into MGPCs. Increasing levels of eCBs through intravitreal injections or upregulation of 2-AG via enzyme inhibitors increased numbers of proliferating MGPCs. Surprisingly, cell death and microglia reactivity were largely unaffected by experimental manipulation of levels eCBs. These data support recent evidence that inflammatory signaling play a pivotal role in regulating reactive gliosis, promoting the de-differentiation in MG, and suppressing the neurogenic capacity of MGPCs.

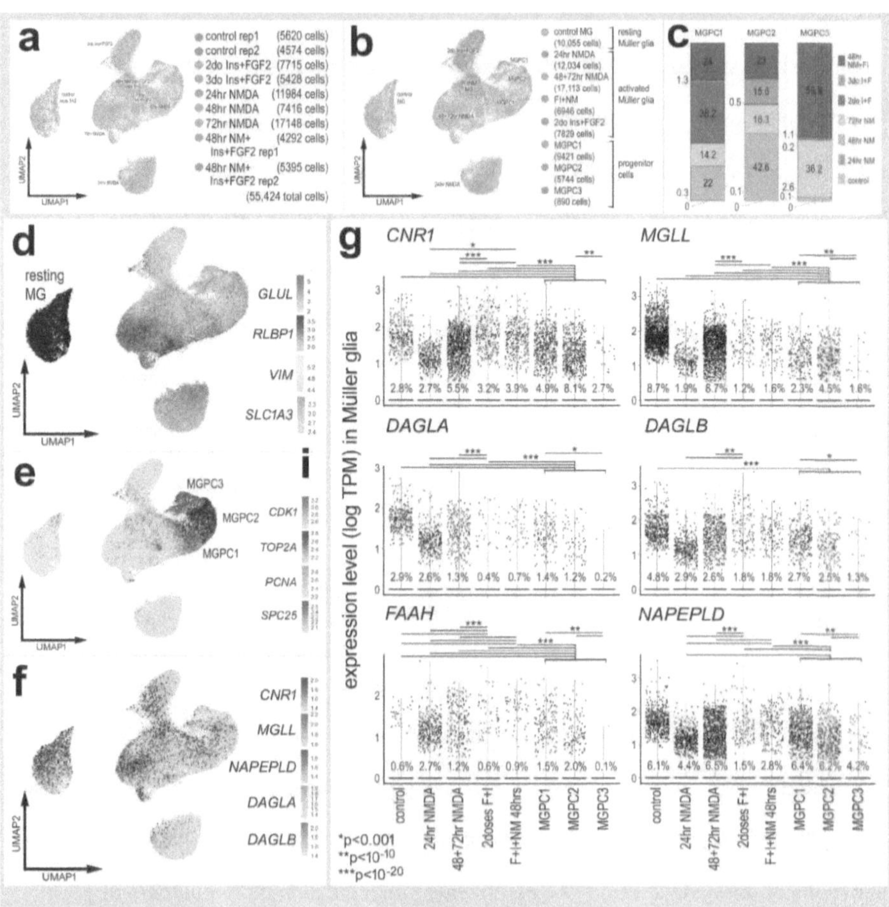

Figure 4.1. MG express genes in the signaling and synthesis of eCBs. scRNA-seq was used to identify patterns of expression of eCB genes in MG at several time points after NMDA damage or FGF + insulin growth factor treatment to form MGPCs. UMAP-clusters of MG were identified by expression of hallmark genes (**a,b,d**). Progenitors were then classified by different cell cycle and progenitor markers (**c, e, f**). Each dot

represents one cell and black dots indicate cells with 2 or more genes expressed. The expression of eCB related genes was illustrated in a colored heatmap and in a violin plot violin plot with population percentages and statistical comparisons. (**g,h,i**). Significant difference (*p<0.01, **p<0.0001, ***p<<0.0001) was determined by using a Wilcox rank sum with Bonferroni correction. MG – Müller glia

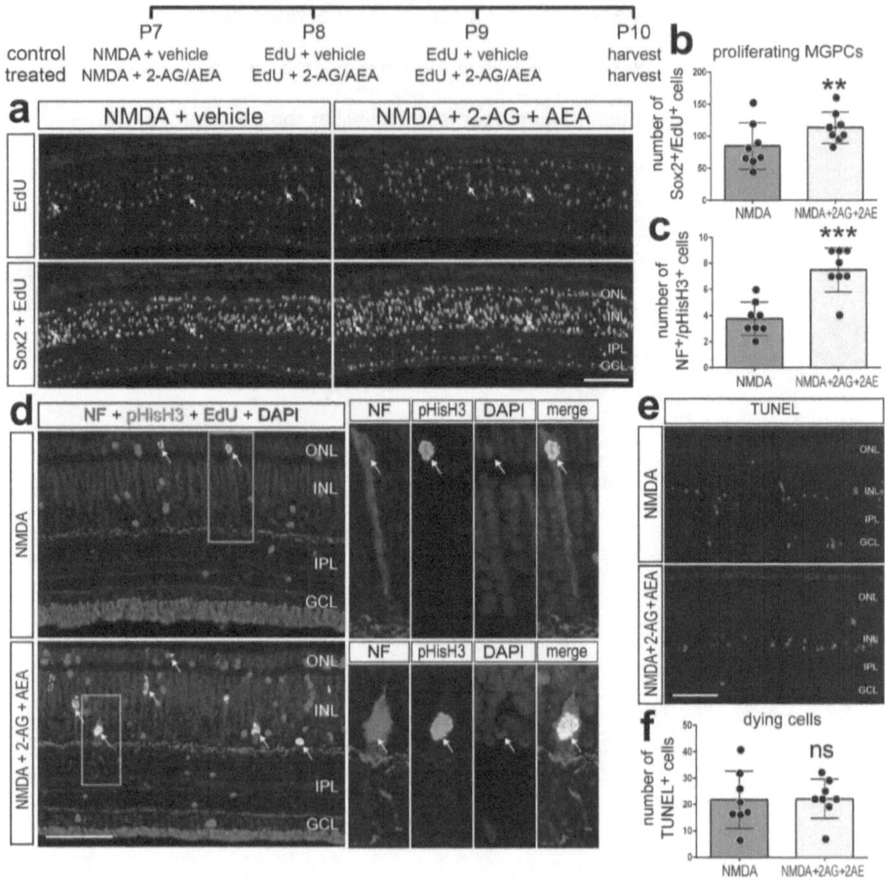

Figure 4.2. eCB injections increase MGPCs after Damage. Chick retinas were injected with the paradigm indicated and detected a measured increase in Sox+ (green) EdU+ (red) cells (**a, c**). Cell death TUNEL assay detected no significant changes in cell death from eCB injections (**b, d**). The transient expression of NF (red) and pHH3 (green) measured actively proliferating cells, which was elevated in the eCB treated retina (**e, f, g**). Each dot represents one biological replicate retina. Significance of

difference (**p<0.01, ***p<0.001) was determined by using a paired *t*-test. Arrows indicate the nuclei of MG. The calibration bar is 50 µm in panels **a, b, e.** Abbreviations: ONL – outer nuclear layer, INL – inner nuclear layer, IPL – inner plexiform layer, GCL – ganglion cell layer.

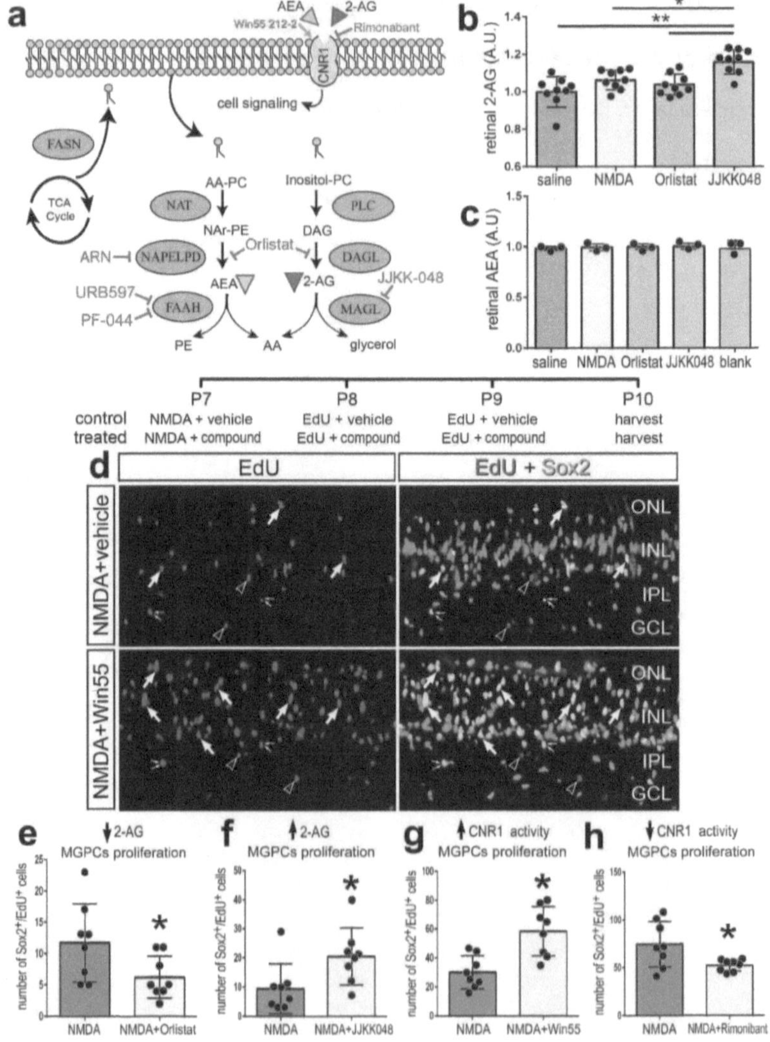

Figure 4.3. Increasing 2-AG signaling pathways with small molecule inhibitors promotes MGPC formation. The presumptive eCB synthesis and signaling pathway

for 2-AG and AEA (**a**). Competitive inhibitor ELISAs of show relative levels of 2-AG and AEA after NMDA damage and inhibitor injection (**b,c**). The representative tissue sections show an increase in Sox2$^+$ (green) and EdU$^+$ (red) MGPCs with inhibitors that boost CNR1 activity (**e, h, i**) and 2-AG signaling (**d, f, g**). The histograms in **b,c,f,g,h,i** represents average quantifications (± SD) and each dot represents one biological replicate retina. The calibration bar in **d** and **e** are 50 µm. Abbreviations: ONL – outer nuclear layer, INL – inner nuclear layer, IPL – inner plexiform layer, GCL – ganglion cell layer.

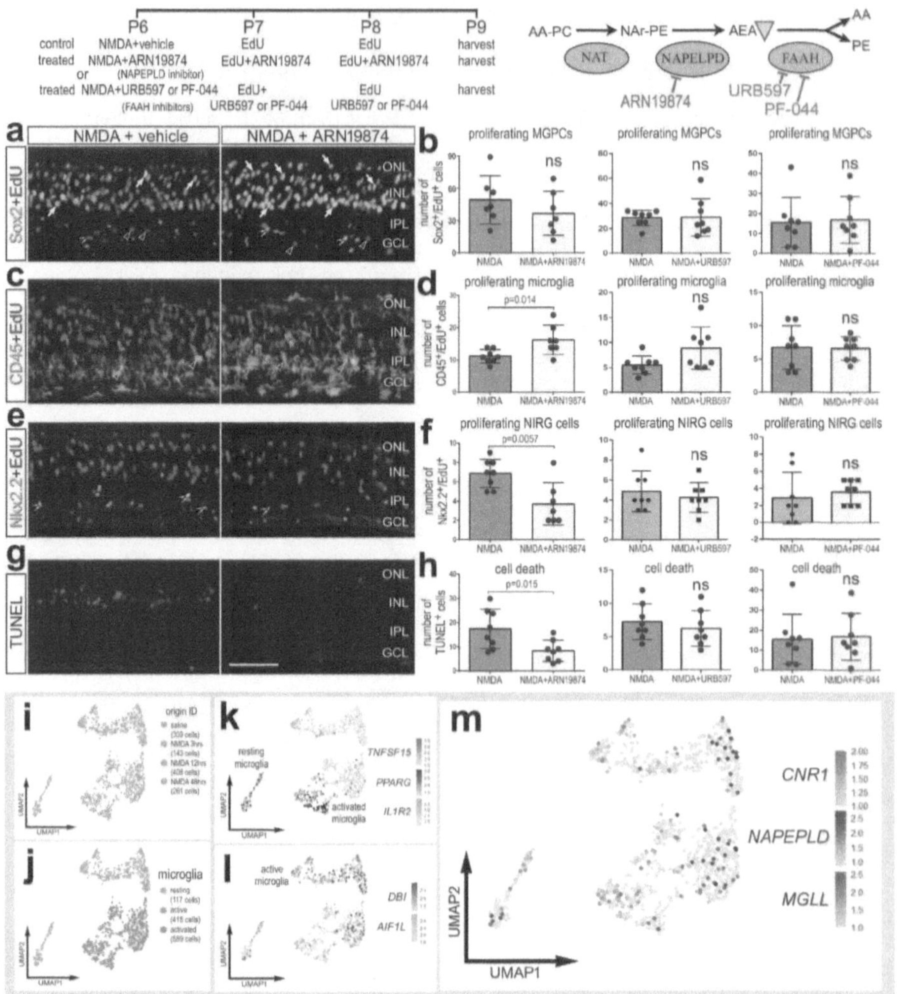

Figure 4.4. Targeting the AEA pathway does not influence MG reprogramming

Inhibitors targeting enzymes in the AEA synthesis pathway were analyzed for their effect on the damaged retina. These drugs did not impact MG reprogramming, as seen by representative Sox2+ (green) and EdU+ (red) MGPCs (**a,b**). The ARN19874 inhibitor did have a marginal effect of increasing microglia proliferation (CD45$^+$ (green) EdU$^+$ (red), **c,d**), NIRG proliferation (Nkx2.2$^+$ (green) EdU$^+$ (red), **e,f**), and cell death (TUNEL$^+$ (red), **g,h**). The FAAH inhibitors had no measurable impact on the retina after damage (**b,d,f,h**). Clusters of microglia isolated from saline and NMDA damaged retinas show no CNR1, but scattered expression of *NAPELPD* and *MGLL* (**i-m**). The histograms in **b,d,f,h** represents average quantifications (± SD) and each dot represents one biological replicate retina. The calibration bar in **g** is 50 µm. Abbreviations: ONL – outer nuclear layer, INL – inner nuclear layer, IPL – inner plexiform layer, GCL – ganglion cell layer.

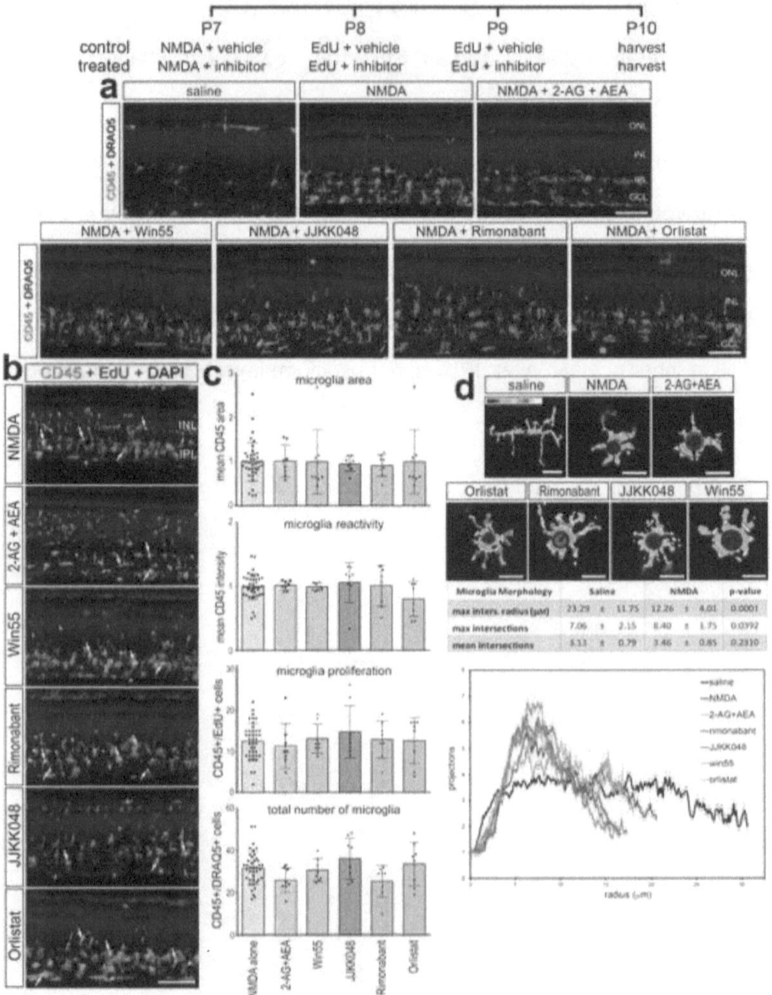

Figure 4.5. Microglia reactivity to retinal damage is unaffected by eCBs

The ramified quiescent microglia become reactive after NMDA damage (a) seen in

representative CD45[+] (green) sections. Microglia reactivity does not significantly change

150

with the addition of eCBs 2-AG and AEA, or small molecule drugs targeting the pathway (control n = 40, treatment n = 8). This includes the area, CD45$^+$ intensity, and total accumulation (**c**). Similarly, the proliferation and accumulation of CD45$^+$ cells are not changed by eCBs or the small molecule inhibitors (**b**). The shape of the microglia was also compared, using a Sholl analysis. Representative microglia from each condition is shown, with a heat map of radial intersections (blue = low, red/white = high) (**c**). A graph of the number of processes radially from the nucleus (±SE) shows the similar shapes among treated microglia (NMDA damage n = 25, undamaged/treatment n = 15) (**d**). Each dot in **c** represents one biological replicate. Significance of difference was determined by using a one-way ANOVA with corresponding Tukey test. The calibration bars panels **a, b** represents 50 µm, and 5µM in **d**. Abbreviations: ONL – outer nuclear layer, INL – inner nuclear layer, IPL – inner plexiform layer, GCL – ganglion cell layer.

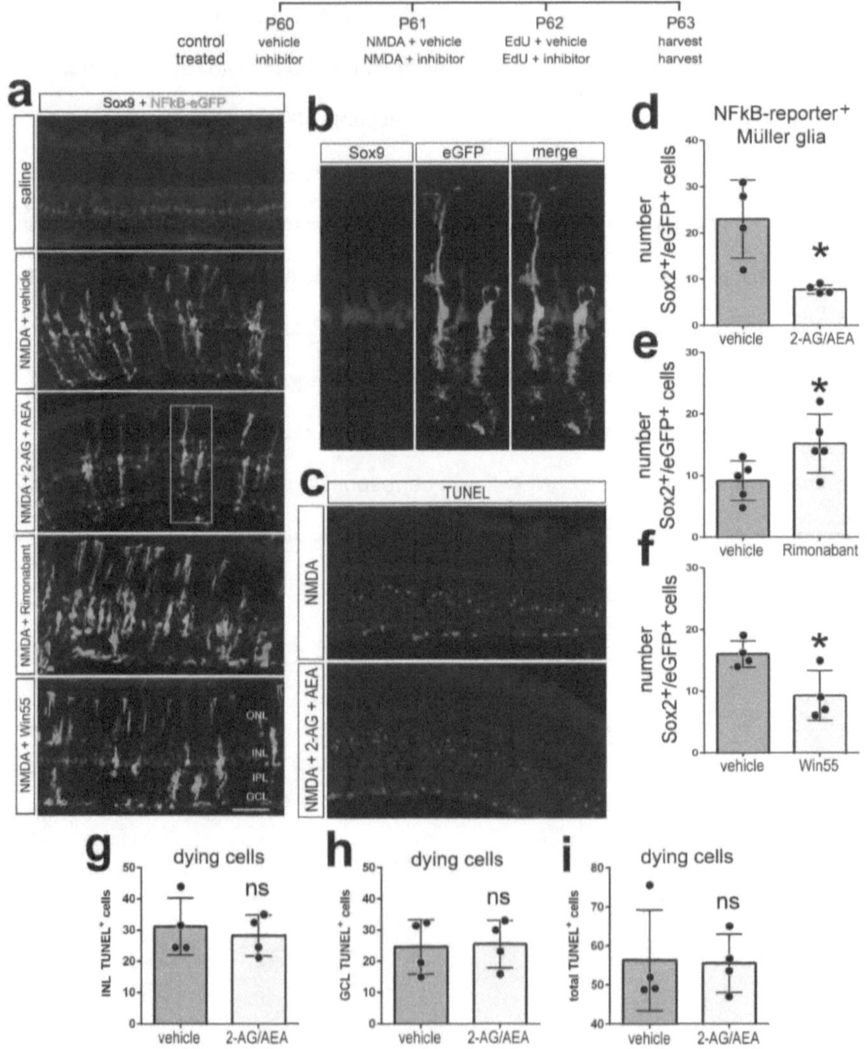

Figure 4.6. eCB reduce NF-kB activation in MG of damaged mouse retina

Mouse retinas of cis-NF-kB[eGFP] were pretreated with eCBs, inhibitor, or saline prior to

damage with NMDA as seen in the schematic. The eGFP+ cells have a MG morphology and Sox2$^+$ nuclei (b). There is a significant reduction in eGFP$^+$ cells with eCB or win55 treatment, where rimonabant treatment significantly increase eGFP$^+$ cells (**a, c, d, e**). the eCBs did not significantly change the number of TUNEL$^+$ dying retinal neurons, either in total or in the INL or GCL layers (**f, g, h, i**). The histogram/scatterplots in **c, d, e, g, h, i** illustrate the mean (±SD) number of labeled cells. Each dot represents one biological replicate. Significance of difference (*p<0.05) was determined by using a paired *t*-test. The calibration bars panels **a, c, e,** and **g** represent 50 µm. Abbreviations: ONL – outer nuclear layer, INL – inner nuclear layer, IPL – inner plexiform layer, GCL – ganglion cell layer.

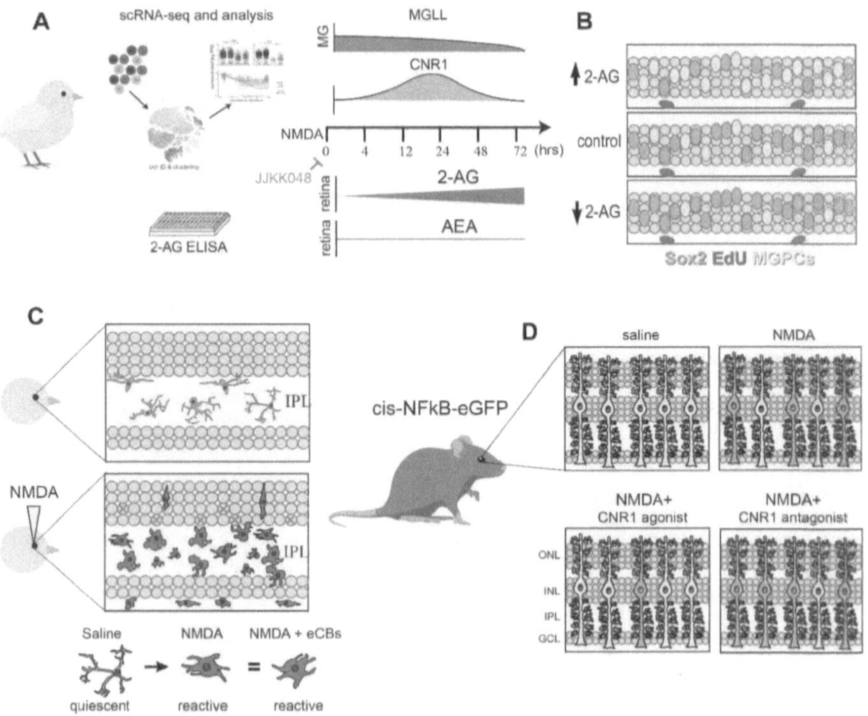

Figure 4.7. Summary Schematic of eCB effect on MG reprogramming. Using scRNA-seq analysis, we denoted the expression and regulation of genes involved in eCB synthesis and signaling (**a**). ELISAs indicated a more prominent role of 2-AG over AEA, and drugs which elevated 2-AG signaling increased MGPCs after damage (**b**). Microglia were unresponsive to these treatments and retained a reactive phenotype in a damaged retina (**c**). In the NF-kBeGFP+ reporter mice, damage activates signaling in MG, which is decreased by exogenous eCBs or CNR1 agonists (**d**).

Table 4.1. Sholl Analysis of chick retinal microglia after damage and eCB drug treatment. Comparative analysis was performed with a one-way Anova and Tukey's test (NMDA n = 25, treatments n = 15)

Microglia Morphology	vehicle	enhance signal			dampen signal		ANOVA
	NMDA	2AG + AEA	JJKK-048	Win55-212,2	Rimonabant	Orlistat	p-value
max inters. radius (μM)	12.26 $\pm$ 4.01	11.90 $\pm$ 3.72	11.99 $\pm$ 3.51	12.65 $\pm$ 5.44	14.01 $\pm$ 5.83	12.27 $\pm$ 2.96	0.782
mean intersections	8.40 $\pm$ 1.75	7.93 $\pm$ 1.83	8.80 $\pm$ 2.54	7.40 $\pm$ 1.76	8.20 $\pm$ 1.85	9.13 $\pm$ 1.88	0.189
max intersections	3.46 $\pm$ 0.85	3.36 $\pm$ 0.61	3.58 $\pm$ 0.86	3.44 $\pm$ 0.81	3.63 $\pm$ 0.70	0.36 $\pm$ 0.68	0.921

Chapter 5

Summary and Future Directions

Synopsis of findings

The data presented in this book focuses on the investigation of factors that contribute to the complex transition from Müller glia to MGPCs in the chick and mouse retina. The data collected via scRNA-seq provided a critical means of leading further inquiry and validation. The data collected primarily investigates the homeostatic dynamics of Müller glia and its proliferative response to injury and growth factor treatment. This work details novel data suggesting that gelatinases, midkine, and eCBs contribute to the reprogramming response of Müller glia.

Chapter two investigates the potential of gelatinases in MGPC formation in the damaged chick retina. MMPs are traditionally known to function in the degradation of the extracellular matrix important for tissue remodeling and cell migration, but also influences cell signaling through the activation of cytokines and growth factor receptors. Glia were the primary source of endogenous retinal gelatinases and other MMPs. While the expression levels were unchanged during reprogramming, the enzymatic activity of gelatinases was depressed, especially in the INL where Müller glia cell bodies are located. This change was observed to be beneficial to reprogramming, and reducing gelatinase activity pharmacologically further boosted the production of MGPCs. The activity decrease correlated with an increase in TIMP2 expression from Müller glia and TIMP3 from NIRG cells. Microglia also contributed to TIMP3 expression, and promoted the production of TIMP3 from NIRGs. This data represents the first data in chick to suggest gelatinases are upstream regulators of MGPC formation.

Chapter two investigates the role midkine in chick and mouse MGPC formation. Midkine is multifunctional and influences the cell cycle, migration, cellular reactivity, and cell growth. Midkine is expressed in developing Müller glia, which is then downregulated in postnatal glia. Damage results in a robust upregulation of midkine for several days after damage or growth factor treatment. Müller glia production has a significant anti-apoptotic effect on NMDA sensitive interneurons. Midkine also had a secondary effect of promoting MGPCs in chick, but this was damage specific and didn't affect growth factor treated retinas. Exogenous administration of midkine resulted in cFos and pS6 upregulation in Müller glia, that was partially blocked through the administration of integrin-B1 signaling inhibitors. These cell signaling changes from midkine administration are conserved in mice, but notably mouse Müller glia do not endogenously express midkine. Exogenous administration of MDK led to a small but significant increase in proliferation of mouse Müller glia when normal NMDA damage results in no MGPCs.

Chapter three focuses on the role of endocannabinoids on MGPC formation. Several studies have validated the relationship of cytokine signaling and MGPC formation in zebrafish, chick, and mouse where the activated pathways and the timing have an impact on the efficiency of reprogramming. eCBs are a retrograde neurotransmitter that also has anti-inflammatory properties. Single cell sequencing identified a subset of amacrine cells as the primary expressors of cannabinoid receptor 1 (CNR1) in the chick and mouse retina. After damage, MG upregulate the CNR1 receptor and downregulate the degrading enzyme MGLL. In chick, increasing eCBs or CNR1 agonists increased the formation of MGPCs in chick. Interestingly, microglia were devoid of detectable CNR receptors and were unresponsive to any changes to eCB production or CNR agonists. In mouse, Müller glia activate the NFkB signaling pathway after damage. CNR agonists reduce the percentage of Müller glia that activate NFkB. This data is novel evidence of the eCB pathway influences NFkB signaling after damage, and that modifying inflammatory signaling on Müller glia may have a robust capacity to influence reprogramming.

Collectively, the data presented in this book provide evidence of novel factors that serve a participatory role in the signaling pathways necessary for Müller glia to transition into a progenitor cell (Fig. 5.1). Each of these factors has an extensive literature regarding their relationship to inflammatory signaling. These works are not comprehensive in establishing a mechanistic understanding of how these factors feed into other established cell signaling cascades aforementioned in the introduction. Thus, a discussion in advancing our current understanding of their relationship to Müller glia reprogramming will be described. Primarily, each subsection will outline prospective studies pursuing the network of factors outlined in the previous chapters.

Prospective studies for MMP signaling in retinal regeneration

As discussed in chapter 2, MMP signaling was investigated as a factor that influenced MGPC formation in the chick. We also demonstrate that immune cells play a role in controlling the level of gelatinase activity in retinal parenchyma after damage. However, we have not thoroughly investigated what pathways are being impacted by the changes in gelatinase activity in retinal tissue.

TGFβ is a secreted cytokine that remains inactive in the tissue matrix (Penn et al., 2012). Under circumstances of tissue injury where tissue healing and remodeling is activated, gelatinases proteolytically degrade its repressive complex allowing it to effectively bind to its receptor in paracrine signaling. Thus, changing TGFβ signaling is dependent not only on production (mRNA levels), but also proteomic changes affecting protein binding dynamics. TGFβ signaling through smad2/3 was found to decrease in chick MGPCs (Todd et al., 2017), but has been found to be essential zebrafish (Lenkowski et al., 2013; Sharma et al., 2020). Furthermore, gelatinase MMP-9 has been correlated to TGFβ signaling in the zebrafish as well as activation of other stem cell transcription factors such as ascl1 (Stanchfield et al., 2020).

Thus, there is precedent that smad2/3 signaling may be impacted by changes in MMP activity. It is difficult to detect changes of TGFβ in the retina, as accurate antibody binding will look analogous to nonspecific background staining. Global changes in activated TGFβ could be measured in whole retina lysate on a western blot at timepoints after damage and gelatinase inhibition. Total TGFβ as well as the gelatinase digested TGFβ band could be quantified as a fraction of activation. This would determine if total levels of TGFβ or the proportion of active TGFβ have been directly influenced by gelatinase inhibitors. For Müller glia TGFβ signaling, an effective phosphorylated smad antibody would be required to detect cell specific changes. A reliable antibody has been difficult to obtain in the chick model. However, western blot analysis is an alternative approach, where we can use GLAST antibodies to fluorescently cell sort Müller glia, and take protein lysates of cytoplasmic and nuclear fractions to determine changes in either smad2/3 or phospho-smad2/3. This data would strengthen the current hypothesis that that gelatinases are upstream activators of TGFβ which has shown to be inhibitory to MGPC formation in chick.

TNFα changes in MMP inhibited retinas

TNFα is a potent inducer of cellular reactivity and inflammation which has been established to be a relevant factor in zebrafish reprogramming (Conner et al., 2014; Iribarne et al., 2019). Recent evidence as shown zebrafish Müller glia produce MMP-9, which is inhibitory to MGPC production and modulate TNFα levels (Silva et al., 2020). We previously discussed how gelatinases could activate TGFβ, but the inhibitors of tissue matrix metalloproteinases also have additional targets other than gelatinases. TIMP3 has been found to also inhibit ADAM17, also known as TNFα converting enzyme (TACE) (Nagase et al., 2006). We had shown that microglia mediate the expression of TIMP3 from other glial cells, and our scRNA-seq data suggests Müller glia express TACE on their cell surface. It was also recently found that TNFα inhibits MGPC formation in chick (Palazzo et al., 2020a). TIMPs may be mediating an important temporal regulator to change when NFkB is active in Müller glia, thus mediating is beneficial or repressive effects.

With reliable antibodies to TIMP2, TIMP3, and TACE, we may be able to convincingly show colocalization of these factors with 63x magnification confocal microscopy after damage. Similarly, we can take whole retina protein lysates and probe for changes in activated TNFα on western blot under conditions of saline, NMDA damage, and exogenous TIMP2/TIMP3 administration. Similarly, we probe for changes in NFkB signaling via phosphorylated NFkB transcription factors on nuclear sorted Müller glia protein lysates.

Future studies for midkine signaling in retinal regeneration

In chapter three, we demonstrate the midkine (MDK) has a multifactorial role in the damaged chick retina. This included a potent neuroprotective effect as well as an autocrine pro-proliferative function to promote the formation of MGPCs. Further study into these roles in chick and mouse will increase MDK's potential as a translatable therapeutic.

How does MDK promote neuroprotection in neurons?

One of the most robust effects observed in the chick retina was its neuroprotection on interneurons. In undamaged retina, exogenous MDK was capable of inducing immediate early gene cFos in amacrine cells and Müller glia. This effect was also present to some degree in mouse retina. This was localized to a subset of neurons that were calretinin positive. In the chick this population consists of both amacrine and bipolar cells, but this is a different population than the subset of cells that experience neuroprotection. There may be direct and indirect mechanisms involved in mediating this effect. The first steps would be to conduct thorough immunolabelling to extract other characteristics of these neuronal subsets that are protected by MDK administration. This would allow us to run probes in the scRNA-seq databases to find corresponding markers to identify these neuronal subsets and run a systematic screen of other MDK related genes and putative receptors. Furthermore, we could probe for other changes in gene expression of this neuronal subset after damage. Changes in neuron expression from excitotoxic damage is an area largely unexplored in these databases. These procedures could be recapitulated in the chick model as well, where the neuroprotective effects are largely recapitulated.

In mouse, Müller glia do not proliferate after NMDA damage. This is largely believed to be an important step in the regeneration process, because models of Müller glia transdifferentiating would reduce endogenous glial populations which may produce the side effect of glial and retinal dysfunction (Jorstad et al., 2020). There are only a few factors that can lead a sizable pool of MGPCs, either Ascl1 overexpression with damage and trichostatin A (Ueki et al., 2015), or transgenic nondegradable β-catenin (Yao et al., 2018). Only a limited number can form with damage and a pharmacological cocktail of growth factors such as EGF (Wan et al., 2012). However, the ability to generate mouse MGPCs via sole pharmacological treatment without damage has remained evasive. Combinatorial preparations of both growth factors and cytokines may yield promising results. Even though MDK was sufficient for meager MGPC production, a systematic titration of other factors may potentiate this effect.

Potential directions of Cannabinoid signaling in retinal regeneration

In chapter four, we present evidence that cannabinoid signaling in the retina influence MGPC formation. There have been previous studies that characterized components of the eCB signaling pathway in the mouse retina (Schwitzer et al., 2016). eCB receptors in the retina also appears conserved in vertebrate species such as rhesus monkey, mouse, rat, chick, goldfish, and salamander (Straiker et al., 1999b). In addition to functional implications of eCBs as neurotransmitters affecting visual processing, they also have been suggested to be anti-inflammatory through CNR1/2 receptors on microglia (Stella, 2009). We present the first data using scRNA-seq to investigate changes in eCB signaling after damage and how modulation of signaling impacts Müller glia reprogramming into MGPCs. With the eCB system showing many parallels between the chick and mouse model that are conducive to follow up studies.

Are there alterations to the cytokine profile of chick microglia after eCB administration?

We have traditionally measured physiologic metrics of reactivity in the retina. After damage, microglia conform into an ameboid shape, proliferate, and upregulate CD45. There is also an accumulation that occurs, likely through the infiltration of circulating CD45[+] macrophages from the choroid (Fischer et al., 2014b). These metrics are unchanged in eCB treated retinas where agonists, antagonists, or inhibitors of degradation or synthesis were applied. This suggests that they are not the primary cell type responding to changes in cannabinoid signaling. The presence of CNR1 on Müller glia and the changing eCB levels changes the number of MGPCs leading to the hypothesis that Müller glia are responding directly to eCBs rather than an indirect mechanism involving paracrine signaling with microglia.

While the parameters of microglia reactivity were unchanged, this does not exclude the possibility that the secretion profile of microglia cytokines are altered by eCB alterations. An in-vitro approach would be to create a culture of chick microglia and apply eCBs with an inducing agent such as lipopolysaccharide (LPS) and perform a western blot on the supernatant for changes in secreted cytokines. These isolated cells can be isolated and probed for inflammatory (IL-1, TNFα, IL-6, INF-γ), anti-inflammatory

(IL-4, IL-10), or neurotrophin secretion (BDNF, NGF). An experiment to confirm the hypothesis that chick microglia are unchanged by eCBs in the chick retina in an in-vivo model, damaged and eCB treated retinas could be dissociated and sorted for CD45$^+$ cells. The aforementioned markers could be measured via quantitative PCR or creating microglia enriched scRNA-seq library with these unique conditions. This data would help elucidate whether the measured outcomes are due to a more direct or indirect mechanism involving Müller glia and/or microglia.

Cell specific anti-inflammatory targeting

In the chick it has been previously demonstrated that dexamethasone is a potent glucocorticoid agonist that has potent anti-inflammatory effect in the chick retina while also inhibiting MGPC formation (Gallina et al., 2014b). Conversely, pharmacological activation of NFkB signaling also demonstrates inhibitory effects on MGPC formation (Palazzo et al., 2020b). While these results may seem contradictory, this may be due to the differential effects of inflammatory and anti-inflammatory signaling on Müller glia and microglia respectively.

There have been evolving strategies using dendrimer polymers that would allow more cell specific targeting to phagocytic cells such as microglia in the retina and have shown promising pro-reprogramming effects in the zebrafish (Emmerich et al., 2021). When dexamethasone is attached directly to this branch polymer, it prevents its broad lipid-based diffusion, and will be targeted to cells that can update these particles. If applied to the chick retina, it may produce differential effects to dexamethasone alone. This would provide evidence that cell specific activation of these inflammatory pathways may be important for effective reprogramming.

Does cell specific CNR1 knockout result in increased or sustained NFkB activation in

Müller glia?

We show that Müller glia are the primary cell type that activate NFkB in the mouse retina after NMDA damage, and that the this can be influenced by targeting CNR1 with agonists and antagonists. Unlike the chick model, we can utilize the transgenic models that exist for CNR1 mice (Marsicano et al., 2003) to study the role of eCB signaling on Müller glia.

We can utilize the CNR1$^{fl/fl}$ floxed mice to ablate CNR1 expression. This can be crossed on cell specific promoters driving cre to get cell specific knockouts in Müller glia (CNR1$^{fl/fl}$ RLBP-ERCre) or in microglia (CNR$^{fl/fl}$ CX3CR1-ERCre). These mice could then be crossed on to the NFkB-GFP reporter mice and measure changes in the number of Müller glia that activate NFkB and the duration of NFkB activity. These experiments would give more cell specific understanding of how this eCB signaling is modifying NFkB in Müller glia through direct or indirect mechanisms.

There has been recent papers showing the importance of microglia in the Ascl1 overexpressing mice in the process of neurogenesis (Todd et al., 2020). This again suggested that even when de-differentiation is forced through Ascl1 overexpression, the presence of microglia signaling to Müller glia have a measurable effect on the complete process of reprogramming. It may yield interesting results to cross the CNR1 floxed mice to the Ascl1 overexpressing mice to see if there are any changes in neurogenesis.

Current state of retinal regeneration research and advancing therapeutic potential

The observation that lower vertebrates could regenerate retinal tissue and restore function has been known since the mid-20th century. In the turn of the 21st century, the field discovered that Müller glia are the source of progenitor cells that regenerate the lost neurons after damage. In the past two decades, dozens of cell signaling pathways have been analyzed for their influence on de-differentiation of Müller glia into MGPCs. was discovered (Gallina et al., 2014a). Some of these approaches have been successfully translated into the mouse model, where transgenic expression models (Jorstad et al., 2017) or AAV delivery models (Yao et al., 2018) can produce some MGPCs. However, this is always in the context of retinal damage, and for this method of neural replacement to be viable, progenitors need to be formed without a concomitant neurotoxic insult and cell death.

The chick model has provided valuable insight into the extrinsic drivers of MGPC reprogramming through paracrine and autocrine signaling factors. This model also provided some of the earliest evidence that Müller glia are the source of regenerated neurons (Fischer and Reh, 2001). While there are many advantages of chick retina, the future of chick research may be restricted by transgenic limitations widely available in mice. Many of the signaling cascades converge on transcription factors that can not be easily targeted pharmacologically. To advance the utility of this model moving forward, utilizing gene editing tools such as Tol2 recombinases (Kawakami, 2007, 2) and CRISPR gene editing (Morin et al., 2017) need to be more widely adapted in chick embryo. We have made advancements in performing embryonic retinal injections that would permit transgene integration in the postnatal chick. This technique bypasses the regulatory and containment overhead of having to house and breed chickens. This will ensure that chick studies will continue to be a versatile model as mouse models advance.

In the mouse, a large factor in the differential effects of cell signaling pathway between species may be the base state chromatin architecture between species. Various deep-sequencing (Norrie et al., 2019) and chromatin immunoprecipitation sequencing (Aldiri et al., 2017; Zibetti et al., 2019) have established important differences during development and neuronal specification. Jak-stat signaling pathways also influence the accessible regions of the chromatin and alter the localization of Ascl1 in mice (Jorstad et al., 2020). With the evolution in scRNA-sequencing technology elucidating new dynamics in mRNA expression patterns during development and reprogramming will need to be more thoroughly applied to the epigenetic landscape of dividing and differentiating cells. To recapitulate the precise coordination of retinal development in reprogrammed cells, these stem cell and pro-neural transcription factors will require a similar chromatin architecture to accurately drive downstream signaling cascades required for neural differentiation. Reprogramming, like development, will require the precise combination of extrinsic and intrinsic stimulation to generate all the different neuronal subtypes in the retina, and more importantly, have these accurately integrate into the appropriate circuits to impact visual perception. Next generation sequencing and single cell multiomics will provide the tools to make more educated hypothesis of the core regulating agents to target in future studies to make this approach more therapeutically viable. However, with the influx of bold claims of regenerated neurons (Blackshaw and Sanes, 2021) with potentially flawed methodology, it is important to conduct these studies methodically including histology, electron microscopy, electrophysiology, and visual function experiments to verify the validity of the most promising approaches. The most robust models should also incorporate Designer Receptors Exclusively Activated by Designer Drugs (DREADDs) such that the restorative effect provided by replaced neurons can have an effective "kill switch" and reverse a restorative phenotype. This strong evidence would reinforce the notion that these new neurons are directly integrated into the visual circuits. Overall, with the rapid pace of advancements in understanding and evolving tools for cellular resolution, this approach for restoring vision in retinal disease will improve in efficiency in mammals.

Concluding Remarks

Retinal diseases affect millions of individuals that lack any therapeutic outlet to restore vision after the retinal neurons have died. The process of vertebrate retinal regeneration is robust, and a compendium of information has been collected regarding the origin, timing, signaling cascades, and transcription factors that coordinate the transition of Müller glia to a neuron. However, the process of translating this cellular metamorphosis is still in its infancy in mouse, and has yet to prove robust enough to reliably improve visual function. The data in this book contributes to the body of work that highlights the important immunomodulation in the spaciotemporal regulation of Müller glia reprogramming. Hopefully this work contributes to the future improvement of evolving reprogramming strategies to reverse blindness in humans.

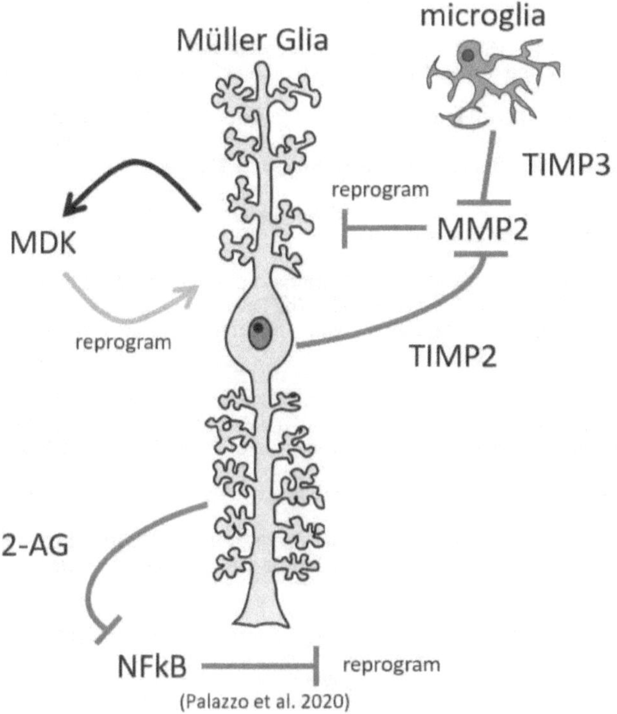

Figure 5.1 Overview of the hypothesized relationships between Müller glia and gelatinase activity, midkine (MDK), and eCBs (2-AG) derived from data presented in this book.

References

Abrams, G. W., Glaser, L. C. (1997). Proliferative vitreoretinopathy. In *Practical atlas of retinal disease and therapy* (ed. Freeman, W. R.), pp. 303–323. Philadelphia: Lippincott-Raven.

Ádám, Á. S., Wenger, T. and Csillag, A. (2008). The cannabinoid CB1 receptor antagonist rimonabant dose-dependently inhibits memory recall in the passive avoidance task in domestic chicks (Gallus domesticus). *Brain Res. Bull.* **76**, 272–274.

Aguzzi, A., Barres, B. A. and Bennett, M. L. (2013). Microglia: Scapegoat, Saboteur, or Something Else? *Science* **339**, 156–161.

Aldiri, I., Xu, B., Wang, L., Chen, X., Hiler, D., Griffiths, L., Valentine, M., Shirinifard, A., Thiagarajan, S., Sablauer, A., et al. (2017). The Dynamic Epigenetic Landscape of the Retina During Development, Reprogramming, and Tumorigenesis. *Neuron* **94**, 550-568.e10.

Ang, N. B., Saera-Vila, A., Walsh, C., Hitchcock, P. F., Kahana, A., Thummel, R. and Nagashima, M. (2020). Midkine-a functions as a universal regulator of proliferation during epimorphic regeneration in adult zebrafish. *PLOS ONE* **15**, e0232308.

Bagrodia, S. and Cerione, R. A. (1999). PAK to the future. *Trends Cell Biol.* **9**, 350–355.

Bernardos, R. L., Barthel, L. K., Meyers, J. R. and Raymond, P. A. (2007). Late-stage neuronal progenitors in the retina are radial Muller glia that function as retinal stem cells. *J Neurosci* **27**, 7028–40.

Bisogno, T., Delton-Vandenbroucke, I., Milone, A., Lagarde, M. and Di Marzo, V. (1999). Biosynthesis and Inactivation of N-Arachidonoylethanolamine (Anandamide) and N-Docosahexaenoylethanolamine in Bovine Retina. *Arch. Biochem. Biophys.* **370**, 300–307.

Bisogno, T., Cascio, M. G., Saha, B., Mahadevan, A., Urbani, P., Minassi, A., Appendino, G., Saturnino, C., Martin, B., Razdan, R., et al. (2006). Development of the first potent and specific inhibitors of endocannabinoid biosynthesis. *Biochim. Biophys. Acta BBA - Mol. Cell Biol. Lipids* **1761**, 205–212.

Blackshaw, S. and Sanes, J. R. (2021). Turning lead into gold: reprogramming retinal cells to cure blindness. *J. Clin. Invest.* **131**,.

Bouskila, J., Javadi, P., Casanova, C., Ptito, M. and Bouchard, J.-F. (2013). Müller cells express the cannabinoid CB2 receptor in the vervet monkey retina. *J. Comp. Neurol.* **521**, 2399–2415.

Bringmann, A. and Reichenbach, A. (2001). Role of Muller cells in retinal degenerations. *Front Biosci* **6**, E72-92.

Bringmann, A., Pannicke, T., Grosche, J., Francke, M., Wiedemann, P., Skatchkov, S. N., Osborne, N. N. and Reichenbach, A. (2006). Müller cells in the healthy and diseased retina. *Prog. Retin. Eye Res.* **25**, 397–424.

Bringmann, A., Iandiev, I., Pannicke, T., Wurm, A., Hollborn, M., Wiedemann, P., Osborne, N. N. and Reichenbach, A. (2009). Cellular signaling and factors involved in Muller cell gliosis: neuroprotective and detrimental effects. *Prog Retin Eye Res* **28**, 423–51.

Brooks, P. C., Strömblad, S., Sanders, L. C., von Schalscha, T. L., Aimes, R. T., Stetler-Stevenson, W. G., Quigley, J. P. and Cheresh, D. A. (1996). Localization of Matrix Metalloproteinase MMP-2 to the Surface of Invasive Cells by Interaction with Integrin αvβ3. *Cell* **85**, 683–693.

Butler, G. S., Butler, M. J., Atkinson, S. J., Will, H., Tamura, T., Westrum, S. S. van, Crabbe, T., Clements, J., d'Ortho, M.-P. and Murphy, G. (1998). The TIMP2 Membrane Type 1 Metalloproteinase "Receptor" Regulates the Concentration and Efficient Activation of Progelatinase A KINETIC STUDY. *J. Biol. Chem.* **273**, 871–880.

Butler, A., Hoffman, P., Smibert, P., Papalexi, E. and Satija, R. (2018). Integrating single-cell transcriptomic data across different conditions, technologies, and species. *Nat. Biotechnol.* **36**, 411–420.

Calinescu, A.-A., Vihtelic, T. S., Hyde, D. R. and Hitchcock, P. F. (2009). The Cellular Expression of Midkine-a and Midkine-b During Retinal Development and Photoreceptor Regeneration in Zebrafish. *J. Comp. Neurol.* **514**, 1–10.

Cameron, D. A. (2000). Cellular proliferation and neurogenesis in the injured retina of adult zebrafish. *Vis Neurosci* **17**, 789–97.

Campbell, W. A., Deshmukh, A., Blum, S., Todd, L., Mendonca, N., Weist, J., Zent, J., Hoang, T. V., Blackshaw, S., Leight, J., et al. (2019). Matrix-metalloproteinase expression and gelatinase activity in the avian retina and their influence on Müller glia proliferation. *Exp. Neurol.* **320**, 112984.

Campbell, W. A., Fritsch-Kelleher, A., Palazzo, I., Hoang, T., Blackshaw, S. and Fischer, A. J. Midkine is neuroprotective and influences glial reactivity and the formation of Müller glia-derived progenitor cells in chick and mouse retinas. *Glia* **n/a**,.

Cawston, T. E., Murphy, G., Mercer, E., Galloway, W. A., Hazleman, B. L. and Reynolds, J. J. (1983). The interaction of purified rabbit bone collagenase with purified rabbit bone metalloproteinase inhibitor. *Biochem. J.* **211**, 313–318.

Centonze, D., Finazzi-Agrò, A., Bernardi, G. and Maccarrone, M. (2007). The endocannabinoid system in targeting inflammatory neurodegenerative diseases. *Trends Pharmacol. Sci.* **28**, 180–187.

Cepko, C. (2014). Intrinsically different retinal progenitor cells produce specific types of progeny. *Nat Rev Neurosci* **15**, 615–27.

Chakraborti, S., Mandal, M., Das, S., Mandal, A. and Chakraborti, T. (2003). Regulation of matrix metalloproteinases: an overview. *Mol. Cell. Biochem.* **253**, 269–285.

Christensen, D. R. G., Brown, F. E., Cree, A. J., Ratnayaka, J. A. and Lotery, A. J. (2017). Sorsby fundus dystrophy – A review of pathology and disease mechanisms. *Exp. Eye Res.* **165**, 35–46.

Clark, B. S., Stein-O'Brien, G. L., Shiau, F., Cannon, G. H., Davis-Marcisak, E., Sherman, T., Santiago, C. P., Hoang, T. V., Rajaii, F., James-Esposito, R. E., et al. (2019). Single-Cell RNA-Seq Analysis of Retinal Development Identifies NFI Factors as Regulating Mitotic Exit and Late-Born Cell Specification. *Neuron* **102**, 1111-1126.e5.

Close, J. L., Liu, J., Gumuscu, B. and Reh, T. A. (2006). Epidermal growth factor receptor expression regulates proliferation in the postnatal rat retina. *Glia* **54**, 94–104.

Common Eye Disorders | Basics | VHI | CDC.

Conner, C., Ackerman, K. M., Lahne, M., Hobgood, J. S. and Hyde, D. R. (2014). Repressing Notch Signaling and Expressing TNFalpha Are Sufficient to Mimic Retinal Regeneration by Inducing Muller Glial Proliferation to Generate Committed Progenitor Cells. *J Neurosci* **34**, 14403–19.

Coulombre, J. L. and Coulombre, A. J. (1965). Regeneration of neural retina from the pigmented epithelium in the chick embryo. *Dev Biol* **12**, 79–92.

da Silva Sampaio, L., Kubrusly, R. C. C., Colli, Y. P., Trindade, P. P., Ribeiro-Resende, V. T., Einicker-Lamas, M., Paes-de-Carvalho, R., Gardino, P. F., de Mello, F. G. and De Melo Reis, R. A. (2018). Cannabinoid Receptor Type 1 Expression in the Developing Avian Retina: Morphological and Functional Correlation With the Dopaminergic System. *Front. Cell. Neurosci.* **12**,.

Dai, L.-C., Yao, X., Wang, X., Niu, S.-Q., Zhou, L.-F., Fu, F.-F., Yang, S.-X. and Ping, J.-L. (2009). In vitro and in vivo suppression of hepatocellular carcinoma growth by midkine-antisense oligonucleotide-loaded nanoparticles. *World J. Gastroenterol. WJG* **15**, 1966–1972.

Dalton, G. D., Bass, C. E., Van Horn, C. and Howlett, A. C. (2009). Signal Transduction via Cannabinoid Receptors. *CNS Neurol. Disord. Drug Targets* **8**, 422–431.

De Luca, A., Maiello, M. R., D'Alessio, A., Pergameno, M. and Normanno, N. (2012). The RAS/RAF/MEK/ERK and the PI3K/AKT signalling pathways: role in cancer pathogenesis and implications for therapeutic approaches. *Expert Opin Ther Targets* **16 Suppl 2**, S17-27.

Deacon, S. W., Beeser, A., Fukui, J. A., Rennefahrt, U. E. E., Myers, C., Chernoff, J. and Peterson, J. R. (2008). An isoform-selective, small-molecule inhibitor targets the autoregulatory mechanism of p21-activated kinase. *Chem. Biol.* **15**, 322–331.

Demb, J. B. and Singer, J. H. (2015). Functional Circuitry of the Retina. *Annu. Rev. Vis. Sci.* **1**, 263–289.

Derouiche, A. and Rauen, T. (1995). Coincidence of L-glutamate/L-aspartate transporter (GLAST) and glutamine synthetase (GS) immunoreactions in retinal glia: evidence for coupling of GLAST and GS in transmitter clearance. *J Neurosci Res* **42**, 131–43.

Diana, M. A. and Bregestovski, P. (2005). Calcium and endocannabinoids in the modulation of inhibitory synaptic transmission. *Cell Calcium* **37**, 497–505.

Dyer, M. A. and Cepko, C. L. (2000). Control of Muller glial cell proliferation and activation following retinal injury. *Nat Neurosci* **3**, 873–80.

Eastlake, K., Banerjee, P. J., Angbohang, A., Charteris, D. G., Khaw, P. T. and Limb, G. A. (2016). Müller glia as an important source of cytokines and inflammatory factors present in the gliotic retina during proliferative vitreoretinopathy. *Glia* **64**, 495–506.

Emmerich, K. B., White, D. T., Kambhampati, S. P., Lee, G. Y., Fu, T.-M., Sahoo, A., Saxena, M. T., Betzig, E., Kannan, R. M. and Mumm, J. S. (2021). Dendrimer-targeted immunosuppression of microglia reactivity super-accelerates photoreceptor regeneration kinetics in the zebrafish retina. *bioRxiv* 2020.08.05.238352.

Emmert-Buck, M. R., Emonard, H., Corcoran, M. L., Krutzsch, H. C., Foidart, J.-M. and Stetler-Stevenson, W. G. (1995). Cell surface binding of TIMP-2 and pro-MMP-2/TIMP-2 complex. *FEBS Lett.* **364**, 28–32.

Fabri, L., Maruta, H., Muramatsu, H., Muramatsu, T., Simpson, R. J., Burgess, A. W. and Nice, E. C. (1993). Structural characterisation of native and recombinant forms of the neurotrophic cytokine MK. *J. Chromatogr.* **646**, 213–225.

Faillace, M. P., Julian, D. and Korenbrot, J. I. (2002). Mitotic activation of proliferative cells in the inner nuclear layer of the mature fish retina: regulatory signals and molecular markers. *J Comp Neurol* **451**, 127–41.

Fairbanks, B. D., Schwartz, M. P., Halevi, A. E., Nuttelman, C. R., Bowman, C. N. and Anseth, K. S. (2009). A Versatile Synthetic Extracellular Matrix Mimic via Thiol-Norbornene Photopolymerization. *Adv. Mater. Deerfield Beach Fla* **21**, 5005–5010.

Fausett, B. V. and Goldman, D. (2006). A role for alpha1 tubulin-expressing Muller glia in regeneration of the injured zebrafish retina. *J Neurosci* **26**, 6303–13.

Fausett, B. V., Gumerson, J. D. and Goldman, D. (2008). The proneural basic helix-loop-helix gene ascl1a is required for retina regeneration. *J. Neurosci. Off. J. Soc. Neurosci.* **28**, 1109–1117.

Fawcett, J. W. and Asher, Richard. A. (1999). The glial scar and central nervous system repair. *Brain Res. Bull.* **49**, 377–391.

Fischer, A. J. (2005). Neural regeneration in the chick retina. *Prog. Retin. Eye Res.* **24**, 161–182.

Fischer, A. J. and Bongini, R. (2010). Turning Müller Glia into Neural Progenitors in the Retina. *Mol. Neurobiol.* **42**, 199–209.

Fischer, A. J. and Reh, T. A. (2000). Identification of a proliferating marginal zone of retinal progenitors in postnatal chickens. *Dev Biol* **220**, 197–210.

Fischer, A. J. and Reh, T. A. (2001). Müller glia are a potential source of neural regeneration in the postnatal chicken retina. *Nat. Neurosci.* **4**, 247–252.

Fischer, A. J. and Reh, T. A. (2002). Exogenous growth factors stimulate the regeneration of ganglion cells in the chicken retina. *Dev Biol* **251**, 367–79.

Fischer, A. J. and Reh, T. A. (2003). Potential of Muller glia to become neurogenic retinal progenitor cells. *Glia* **43**, 70–6.

Fischer, A. J., Seltner, R. L. P., Poon, J. and Stell, W. K. (1998). Immunocytochemical characterization of quisqualic acid- and N-methyl-D-aspartate-induced excitotoxicity in the retina of chicks. *J. Comp. Neurol.* **393**, 1–15.

Fischer, A. J., Dierks, B. D. and Reh, T. A. (2002a). Exogenous growth factors induce the production of ganglion cells at the retinal margin. *Development* **129**, 2283–91.

Fischer, A. J., McGuire, C. R., Dierks, B. D. and Reh, T. A. (2002b). Insulin and Fibroblast Growth Factor 2 Activate a Neurogenic Program in Müller Glia of the Chicken Retina. *J. Neurosci.* **22**, 9387–9398.

Fischer, A. J., Schmidt, M., Omar, G. and Reh, T. A. (2004). BMP4 and CNTF are neuroprotective and suppress damage-induced proliferation of Muller glia in the retina. *Mol Cell Neurosci* **27**, 531–42.

Fischer, A. J., Foster, S., Scott, M. A. and Sherwood, P. (2008). The transient expression of LIM-domain transcription factors is coincident with the delayed maturation of photoreceptors in the chicken retina. *J. Comp. Neurol.* **506**, 584–603.

Fischer, A. J., Scott, M. A., Ritchey, E. R. and Sherwood, P. (2009a). Mitogen-activated protein kinase-signaling regulates the ability of Müller glia to proliferate and protect retinal neurons against excitotoxicity. *Glia* **57**, 1538–1552.

Fischer, A. J., Scott, M. A. and Tuten, W. (2009b). Mitogen-activated protein kinase-signaling stimulates Müller glia to proliferate in acutely damaged chicken retina. *Glia* **57**, 166–181.

Fischer, A. J., Scott, M. A., Zelinka, C. and Sherwood, P. (2010). A novel type of glial cell in the retina is stimulated by insulin-like growth factor 1 and may exacerbate damage to neurons and Muller glia. *Glia* **58**, 633–49.

Fischer, A. J., Zelinka, C., Gallina, D., Scott, M. A. and Todd, L. (2014a). Reactive microglia and macrophage facilitate the formation of Muller glia-derived retinal progenitors. *Glia* **62**, 1608–28.

Fischer, A. J., Zelinka, C., Gallina, D., Scott, M. A. and Todd, L. (2014b). Reactive microglia and macrophage facilitate the formation of Müller glia-derived retinal progenitors. *Glia* **62**, 1608–1628.

Fischer, A. J., Zelinka, C. and Milani-Nejad, N. (2015). Reactive retinal microglia, neuronal survival, and the formation of retinal folds and detachments. *Glia* **63**, 313–27.

Fitch, J. M., Kidder, J. M. and Linsenmayer, T. F. (2005). Cellular invasion of the chicken corneal stroma during development: Regulation by multiple matrix metalloproteases and the lens. *Dev. Dyn.* **232**, 106–118.

Frampton, G., Coufal, M., Li, H., Ramirez, J. and DeMorrow, S. (2010). Opposing actions of endocannabinoids on cholangiocarcinoma growth is via the differential activation of Notch signaling. *Exp. Cell Res.* **316**, 1465–1478.

Frisch, S. M. (2000). cAMP takes control. *Nat. Cell Biol.* **2**, E167–E168.

Fu, X., Zhu, J., Duan, Y., Li, G., Cai, H., Zheng, L., Qian, H., Zhang, C., Jin, Z., Fu, X.-D., et al. (2020). Visual function restoration in genetically blind mice via endogenous cellular reprogramming. *bioRxiv* 2020.04.08.030981.

Fujikawa, A., Nagahira, A., Sugawara, H., Ishii, K., Imajo, S., Matsumoto, M., Kuboyama, K., Suzuki, R., Tanga, N., Noda, M., et al. (2016). Small-molecule inhibition of PTPRZ reduces tumor growth in a rat model of glioblastoma. *Sci. Rep.* **6**, 20473.

Fukada, M., Fujikawa, A., Chow, J. P. H., Ikematsu, S., Sakuma, S. and Noda, M. (2006). Protein tyrosine phosphatase receptor type Z is inactivated by ligand-induced oligomerization. *FEBS Lett.* **580**, 4051–4056.

Gallina, D. Z., C. P. Cebulla, C. M. Fischer, A. J. (2015). Activation of glucocorticoid receptors in Müller glia is protective to retinal neurons and suppresses microglial reactivity. *Exp Neurol* **273**, 114–125.

Gallina, D., Todd, L. and Fischer, A. J. (2014a). A comparative analysis of Müller glia-mediated regeneration in the vertebrate retina. *Exp. Eye Res.* **123**, 121–130.

Gallina, D., Zelinka, C. and Fischer, A. J. (2014b). Glucocorticoid receptors in the retina, Muller glia and the formation of Muller glia-derived progenitors. *Development* **141**, 3340–51.

Gallina, D., Zelinka, C. P., Cebulla, C. and Fischer, A. J. (2015). Activation of glucocorticoid receptors in Müller glia is protective to retinal neurons and suppresses microglial reactivity. *Exp. Neurol.* **273**, 114–125.

Gallina, D., Palazzo, I., Steffenson, L., Todd, L. and Fischer, A. J. (2016). Wnt/β-catenin-signaling and the formation of Müller glia-derived progenitors in the chick retina. *Dev. Neurobiol.* **76**, 983–1002.

Ghai, K., Zelinka, C. and Fischer, A. J. (2009). Serotonin released from amacrine neurons is scavenged and degraded in bipolar neurons in the retina. *J Neurochem* **111**, 1–14.

Ghai, K., Zelinka, C. and Fischer, A. J. (2010). Notch signaling influences neuroprotective and proliferative properties of mature Muller glia. *J Neurosci* **30**, 3101–12.

Gilbert, C. and Foster, A. (2001). Childhood blindness in the context of VISION 2020--the right to sight. *Bull. World Health Organ.* **79**, 227–232.

Ginhoux, F., Greter, M., Leboeuf, M., Nandi, S., See, P., Gokhan, S., Mehler, M. F., Conway, S. J., Ng, L. G., Stanley, E. R., et al. (2010). Fate mapping analysis reveals that adult microglia derive from primitive macrophages. *Science* **330**, 841–5.

Goldman, D. (2014). Müller glial cell reprogramming and retina regeneration. *Nat. Rev. Neurosci.* **15**, 431–442.

Gramage, E., Li, J. and Hitchcock, P. (2014). The expression and function of midkine in the vertebrate retina. *Br J Pharmacol* **171**, 913–23.

Gramage, E., D'Cruz, T., Taylor, S., Thummel, R. and Hitchcock, P. F. (2015). Midkine-a Protein Localization in the Developing and Adult Retina of the Zebrafish and Its Function During Photoreceptor Regeneration. *PLoS ONE* **10**,.

Hamburger, V., Hamilton, HL (1951). A series of normal stages in the development of the chick embryo. *J. Morphol.* **88**, 49–92.

Hao, H., Maeda, Y., Fukazawa, T., Yamatsuji, T., Takaoka, M., Bao, X.-H., Matsuoka, J., Okui, T., Shimo, T., Takigawa, N., et al. (2013). Inhibition of the Growth Factor MDK/Midkine by a Novel Small Molecule Compound to Treat Non-Small Cell Lung Cancer. *PLOS ONE* **8**, e71093.

Hayes, S., Nelson, B. R., Buckingham, B. and Reh, T. A. (2007). Notch signaling regulates regeneration in the avian retina. *Dev Biol* **312**, 300–11.

Hehr, C. L., Hocking, J. C. and McFarlane, S. (2005). Matrix metalloproteinases are required for retinal ganglion cell axon guidance at select decision points. *Development* **132**, 3371–3379.

Hickey, D. G., Edwards, T. L., Barnard, A. R., Singh, M. S., Silva, S. R. de, McClements, M. E., Flannery, J. G., Hankins, M. W. and MacLaren, R. E. (2017). Tropism of engineered and evolved recombinant AAV serotypes in the rd1 mouse and ex vivo primate retina. *Gene Ther.* **24**, 787.

Hienola, A., Pekkanen, M., Raulo, E., Vanttola, P. and Rauvala, H. (2004). HB-GAM inhibits proliferation and enhances differentiation of neural stem cells. *Mol. Cell. Neurosci.* **26**, 75–88.

Hillard, C. J. (2015). The Endocannabinoid Signaling System in the CNS. In *International Review of Neurobiology*, pp. 1–47. Elsevier.

Hippert, C., Graca, A. B., Barber, A. C., West, E. L., Smith, A. J., Ali, R. R. and Pearson, R. A. (2015). Müller Glia Activation in Response to Inherited Retinal Degeneration Is Highly Varied and Disease-Specific. *PLOS ONE* **10**, e0120415.

Hitchcock, P. F. (1997). Tracer coupling among regenerated amacrine cells in the retina of the goldfish. *Vis Neurosci* **14**, 463–72.

Hitchcock, P. F. and Raymond, P. A. (1992). Retinal regeneration. *Trends Neurosci* **15**, 103–8.

Hoang, T., Wang, J., Boyd, P., Wang, F., Santiago, C., Jiang, L., Yoo, S., Lahne, M., Todd, L. J., Jia, M., et al. (2020). Gene regulatory networks controlling vertebrate retinal regeneration. *Science* **370**,.

Hollborn, M., Tenckhoff, S., Jahn, K., Iandiev, I., Biedermann, B., Schnurrbusch, U. E., Limb, G. A., Reichenbach, A., Wolf, S., Wiedemann, P., et al. (2005). Changes in retinal gene expression in proliferative vitreoretinopathy: glial cell expression of HB-EGF. *Mol Vis* **11**, 397–413.

Horiguchi, M., Ota, M. and Rifkin, D. B. (2012). Matrix control of transforming growth factor-β function. *J. Biochem. (Tokyo)* **152**, 321–329.

Howard, E. W., Bullen, E. C. and Banda, M. J. (1991). Preferential inhibition of 72- and 92-kDa gelatinases by tissue inhibitor of metalloproteinases-2. *J. Biol. Chem.* **266**, 13070–13075.

Hu, S. S.-J., Arnold, A., Hutchens, J. M., Radicke, J., Cravatt, B. F., Wager-Miller, J., Mackie, K. and Straiker, A. (2010). Architecture of cannabinoid signaling in mouse retina. *J. Comp. Neurol.* **518**, 3848–3866.

Ichihara-Tanaka, K., Oohira, A., Rumsby, M. and Muramatsu, T. (2006). Neuroglycan C Is a Novel Midkine Receptor Involved in Process Elongation of Oligodendroglial Precursor-like Cells. *J. Biol. Chem.* **281**, 30857–30864.

Ihanamäki, T., Pelliniemi, L. J. and Vuorio, E. (2004). Collagens and collagen-related matrix components in the human and mouse eye. *Prog. Retin. Eye Res.* **23**, 403–434.

Inoue, M., Nakayama, C. and Noguchi, H. (1996). Activating mechanism of CNTF and related cytokines. *Mol Neurobiol* **12**, 195–209.

Iribarne, M., Hyde, D. R. and Masai, I. (2019). TNFα Induces Müller Glia to Transition From Non-proliferative Gliosis to a Regenerative Response in Mutant Zebrafish Presenting Chronic Photoreceptor Degeneration. *Front. Cell Dev. Biol.* **7**,.

Islam, S., Zeisel, A., Joost, S., La Manno, G., Zajac, P., Kasper, M., Lönnerberg, P. and Linnarsson, S. (2014). Quantitative single-cell RNA-seq with unique molecular identifiers. *Nat. Methods* **11**, 163–166.

Itoh, Y., Ito, A., Iwata, K., Tanzawa, K., Mori, Y. and Nagase, H. (1998). Plasma Membrane-bound Tissue Inhibitor of Metalloproteinases (TIMP)-2 Specifically Inhibits Matrix Metalloproteinase 2 (Gelatinase A) Activated on the Cell Surface. *J. Biol. Chem.* **273**, 24360–24367.

Ivaska, J., Reunanen, H., Westermarck, J., Koivisto, L., Kähäri, V.-M. and Heino, J. (1999). Integrin α2β1 Mediates Isoform-Specific Activation of p38 and Upregulation of Collagen Gene Transcription by a Mechanism Involving the α2 Cytoplasmic Tail. *J. Cell Biol.* **147**, 401–416.

Ivaska, J., Nissinen, L., Immonen, N., Eriksson, J. E., Kähäri, V.-M. and Heino, J. (2002). Integrin α2β1 Promotes Activation of Protein Phosphatase 2A and Dephosphorylation of Akt and Glycogen Synthase Kinase 3β. *Mol. Cell. Biol.* **22**, 1352–1359.

Iwasaki, W., Nagata, K., Hatanaka, H., Inui, T., Kimura, T., Muramatsu, T., Yoshida, K., Tasumi, M. and Inagaki, F. (1997). Solution structure of midkine, a new heparin-binding growth factor. *EMBO J.* **16**, 6936–6946.

Iyer, R. P., Patterson, N. L., Fields, G. B. and Lindsey, M. L. (2012). The history of matrix metalloproteinases: milestones, myths, and misperceptions. *Am. J. Physiol. - Heart Circ. Physiol.* **303**, H919–H930.

Jayaram, H., Jones, M. F., Eastlake, K., Cottrill, P. B., Becker, S., Wiseman, J., Khaw, P. T. and Limb, G. A. (2014). Transplantation of photoreceptors derived from human Muller glia restore rod function in the P23H rat. *Stem Cells Transl Med* **3**, 323–33.

Jochheim-Richter, A., Rüdrich, U., Koczan, D., Hillemann, T., Tewes, S., Petry, M., Kispert, A., Sharma, A. D., Attaran, F., Manns, M. P., et al. (2006). Gene expression analysis identifies novel genes participating in early murine liver development and adult liver regeneration. *Differentiation* **74**, 167–173.

John, G. R., Lee, S. C. and Brosnan, C. F. (2003). Cytokines: Powerful Regulators of Glial Cell Activation. *The Neuroscientist* **9**, 10–22.

Jorstad, N. L., Wilken, M. S., Grimes, W. N., Wohl, S. G., VandenBosch, L. S., Yoshimatsu, T., Wong, R. O., Rieke, F. and Reh, T. A. (2017). Stimulation of functional neuronal regeneration from Muller glia in adult mice. *Nature*.

Jorstad, N. L., Wilken, M. S., Todd, L., Finkbeiner, C., Nakamura, P., Radulovich, N., Hooper, M. J., Chitsazan, A., Wilkerson, B. A., Rieke, F., et al. (2020). STAT Signaling Modifies Ascl1 Chromatin Binding and Limits Neural Regeneration from Muller Glia in Adult Mouse Retina. *Cell Rep.* **30**, 2195-2208.e5.

Jung, C.-G., Hida, H., Nakahira, K., Ikenaka, K., Kim, H.-J. and Nishino, H. (2004). Pleiotrophin mRNA is highly expressed in neural stem (progenitor) cells of mouse ventral mesencephalon and the product promotes production of dopaminergic neurons from embryonic stem cell-derived nestin-positive cells. *FASEB J.* **18**, 1237–1239.

Kang, H. C., Kim, I.-J., Park, J.-H., Shin, Y., Ku, J.-L., Jung, M. S., Yoo, B. C., Kim, H. K. and Park, J.-G. (2004). Identification of Genes with Differential Expression in Acquired Drug-Resistant Gastric Cancer Cells Using High-Density Oligonucleotide Microarrays. *Clin. Cancer Res.* **10**, 272–284.

Karl, M. O. and Reh, T. A. (2010). Regenerative medicine for retinal diseases: activating the endogenous repair mechanisms. *Trends Mol. Med.* **16**, 193–202.

Karl, M. O., Hayes, S., Nelson, B. R., Tan, K., Buckingham, B. and Reh, T. A. (2008). Stimulation of neural regeneration in the mouse retina. *Proc Natl Acad Sci U A* **105**, 19508–13.

Kassen, S. C., Thummel, R., Campochiaro, L. A., Harding, M. J., Bennett, N. A. and Hyde, D. R. (2009). CNTF induces photoreceptor neuroprotection and Muller glial cell proliferation through two different signaling pathways in the adult zebrafish retina. *Exp Eye Res* **88**, 1051–64.

Kaur, S., Gupta, S., Chaudhary, M., Khursheed, M. A., Mitra, S., Kurup, A. J. and Ramachandran, R. (2018). let-7 MicroRNA-Mediated Regulation of Shh Signaling and the Gene Regulatory Network Is Essential for Retina Regeneration. *Cell Rep.* **23**, 1409–1423.

Kawachi, H., Fujikawa, A., Maeda, N. and Noda, M. (2001). Identification of GIT1/Cat-1 as a substrate molecule of protein tyrosine phosphatase ζ/β by the yeast substrate-trapping system. *Proc. Natl. Acad. Sci. U. S. A.* **98**, 6593–6598.

Kawakami, K. (2007). Tol2: a versatile gene transfer vector in vertebrates. *Genome Biol.* **8**, S7.

Kawasaki, T. and Kawai, T. (2014). Toll-Like Receptor Signaling Pathways. *Front. Immunol.* **5**,.

Kikuchi-Horie, K., Kawakami, E., Kamata, M., Wada, M., Hu, J.-G., Nakagawa, H., Ohara, K., Watabe, K. and Oyanagi, K. (2004). Distinctive expression of midkine in the repair period of rat brain during neurogenesis: Immunohistochemical and immunoelectron microscopic observations. *J. Neurosci. Res.* **75**, 678–687.

Kilpeläinen, I., Kaksonen, M., Kinnunen, §‖ Tarja, Avikainen, H., Fath, M., Linhardt, R. J., Raulo, E. and Rauvala, H. (2000). Heparin-binding Growth-associated Molecule Contains Two Heparin-binding β-Sheet Domains That Are Homologous to the Thrombospondin Type I Repeat. *J. Biol. Chem.* **275**, 13564–13570.

Kim, S.-M., Kwon, M. S., Park, C. S., Choi, K.-R., Chun, J.-S., Ahn, J. and Song, W. K. (2004). Modulation of Thr Phosphorylation of Integrin β1 during Muscle Differentiation. *J. Biol. Chem.* **279**, 7082–7090.

Kohsaka, S., Takamatsu, K., Nishimura, Y., Mikoshiba, K. and Tsukada, Y. (1980). Neurochemical characteristics of myelin-like structure in the chick retina. *J Neurochem* **34**, 662–8.

Kojima, T., Katsumi, A., Yamazaki, T., Muramatsu, T., Nagasaka, T., Ohsumi, K. and Saito, H. (1996). Human Ryudocan from Endothelium-like Cells Binds Basic Fibroblast Growth Factor, Midkine, and Tissue Factor Pathway Inhibitor. *J. Biol. Chem.* **271**, 5914–5920.

Kokona, D., Spyridakos, D., Tzatzarakis, M., Papadogkonaki, S., Filidou, E., Arvanitidis, K. I., Kolios, G., Lamani, M., Makriyannis, A., Malamas, M. S., et al. (2021). The endocannabinoid 2-arachidonoylglycerol and dual ABHD6/MAGL enzyme inhibitors display neuroprotective and anti-inflammatory actions in the in vivo retinal model of AMPA excitotoxicity. *Neuropharmacology* **185**, 108450.

Könnecke, H. and Bechmann, I. (2013). The Role of Microglia and Matrix Metalloproteinases Involvement in Neuroinflammation and Gliomas. *J. Immunol. Res.*

Kridel, S. J., Axelrod, F., Rozenkrantz, N. and Smith, J. W. (2004). Orlistat Is a Novel Inhibitor of Fatty Acid Synthase with Antitumor Activity. *Cancer Res.* **64**, 2070–2075.

Kuboyama, K., Fujikawa, A., Suzuki, R. and Noda, M. (2015). Inactivation of Protein Tyrosine Phosphatase Receptor Type Z by Pleiotrophin Promotes Remyelination through Activation of Differentiation of Oligodendrocyte Precursor Cells. *J. Neurosci.* **35**, 12162–12171.

Kumar, A. and Shamsuddin, N. (2012). Retinal Muller Glia Initiate Innate Response to Infectious Stimuli via Toll-Like Receptor Signaling. *PLOS ONE* **7**, e29830.

Kumar, R., Gururaj, A. E. and Barnes, C. J. (2006). p21-activated kinases in cancer. *Nat. Rev. Cancer* **6**, 459.

Kumar, A., Pandey, R. K., Miller, L. J., Singh, P. K. and Kanwar, M. (2013). Müller Glia in Retinal Innate Immunity: A perspective on their roles in endophthalmitis. *Crit. Rev. Immunol.* **33**, 119–135.

Kurosawa, N., Chen, G.-Y., Kadomatsu, K., Ikematsu, S., Sakuma, S. and Muramatsu, T. (2001). Glypican-2 binds to midkine: The role of glypican-2 in neuronal cell adhesion and neurite outgrowth. *Glycoconj. J.* **18**, 499–507.

Laferriere, N. B., MacRae, T. H. and Brown, D. L. (1997). Tubulin synthesis and assembly in differentiating neurons. *Biochem Cell Biol* **75**, 103–17.

Leight, J. L., Alge, D. L., Maier, A. J. and Anseth, K. S. (2013). Direct measurement of matrix metalloproteinase activity in 3D cellular microenvironments using a fluorogenic peptide substrate. *Biomaterials* **34**, 7344–7352.

Lenkowski, J. R., Qin, Z., Sifuentes, C. J., Thummel, R., Soto, C. M., Moens, C. B. and Raymond, P. A. (2013). Retinal regeneration in adult zebrafish requires regulation of TGFbeta signaling. *Glia* **61**, 1687–97.

Liddelow, S. A., Guttenplan, K. A., Clarke, L. E., Bennett, F. C., Bohlen, C. J., Schirmer, L., Bennett, M. L., Munch, A. E., Chung, W. S., Peterson, T. C., et al. (2017). Neurotoxic reactive astrocytes are induced by activated microglia. *Nature* **541**, 481–487.

Lin, X. (2004). Functions of heparan sulfate proteoglycans in cell signaling during development. *Development* **131**, 6009–6021.

Liu, Y., Beyer, A. and Aebersold, R. (2016). On the Dependency of Cellular Protein Levels on mRNA Abundance. *Cell* **165**, 535–550.

Liu, T., Zhang, L., Joo, D. and Sun, S.-C. (2017). NF-κB signaling in inflammation. *Signal Transduct. Target. Ther.* **2**, 17023.

Livesey, F. J. and Cepko, C. L. (2001). Vertebrate neural cell-fate determination: lessons from the retina. *Nat Rev Neurosci* **2**, 109–18.

Llano, E., Pendás, A. M., Freije, J. P., Nakano, A., Knäuper, V., Murphy, G. and López-Otin, C. (1999). Identification and Characterization of Human MT5-MMP, a New Membrane-bound Activator of Progelatinase A Overexpressed in Brain Tumors. *Cancer Res.* **59**, 2570–2576.

Logan, P., Marshall, J.-C. A., Fernandes, B. F., Bakalian, S., Martins, C. and M. N. Burnier, J. (2007). MMP-2 and MMP-9 Secretion by Human Uveal Melanoma Cell Lines in Response to Different Growth Factors and Chemokines. *Invest. Ophthalmol. Vis. Sci.* **48**, 4766–4766.

Luo, J., Uribe, R. A., Hayton, S., Calinescu, A.-A., Gross, J. M. and Hitchcock, P. F. (2012). Midkine-A functions upstream of Id2a to regulate cell cycle kinetics in the developing vertebrate retina. *Neural Develop.* **7**, 33.

Mader, M. M. and Cameron, D. A. (2004). Photoreceptor differentiation during retinal development, growth, and regeneration in a metamorphic vertebrate. *J Neurosci* **24**, 11463–72.

Maeda, N., Ichihara-Tanaka, K., Kimura, T., Kadomatsu, K., Muramatsu, T. and Noda, M. (1999). A Receptor-like Protein-tyrosine Phosphatase PTPζ/RPTPβ Binds a Heparin-binding Growth Factor Midkine INVOLVEMENT OF ARGININE 78 OF MIDKINE IN THE HIGH AFFINITY BINDING TO PTPζ. *J. Biol. Chem.* **274**, 12474–12479.

Magness, S. T., Jijon, H., Van Houten Fisher, N., Sharpless, N. E., Brenner, D. A. and Jobin, C. (2004). In vivo pattern of lipopolysaccharide and anti-CD3-induced NF-kappa B activation using a novel gene-targeted enhanced GFP reporter gene mouse. *J Immunol* **173**, 1561–70.

Marsicano, G., Goodenough, S., Monory, K., Hermann, H., Eder, M., Cannich, A., Azad, S. C., Cascio, M. G., Gutiérrez, S. O., van der Stelt, M., et al. (2003). CB1 cannabinoid receptors and on-demand defense against excitotoxicity. *Science* **302**, 84–88.

Martin, K., Pritchett, J., Llewellyn, J., Mullan, A. F., Athwal, V. S., Dobie, R., Harvey, E., Zeef, L., Farrow, S., Streuli, C., et al. (2016). PAK proteins and YAP-1 signalling downstream of integrin beta-1 in myofibroblasts promote liver fibrosis. *Nat. Commun.* **7**, 1–11.

Mashima, T., Sato, S., Sugimoto, Y., Tsuruo, T. and Seimiya, H. (2009). Promotion of glioma cell survival by acyl-CoA synthetase 5 under extracellular acidosis conditions. *Oncogene* **28**, 9–19.

Masui, M., Okui, T., Shimo, T., Takabatake, K., Fukazawa, T., Matsumoto, K., Kurio, N., Ibaragi, S., Naomoto, Y., Nagatsuka, H., et al. (2016). Novel Midkine Inhibitor iMDK Inhibits Tumor Growth and Angiogenesis in Oral Squamous Cell Carcinoma. *Anticancer Res.* **36**, 2775–2781.

Matsuda, S., Kanemitsu, N., Nakamura, A., Mimura, Y., Ueda, N., Kurahashi, Y. and Yamamoto, S. (1997). Metabolism of Anandamide, an Endogenous Cannabinoid Receptor Ligand, in Porcine Ocular Tissues. *Exp. Eye Res.* **64**, 707–711.

McInnes, L., Healy, J. and Melville, J. (2018). UMAP: Uniform Manifold Approximation and Projection for Dimension Reduction. *Eprint ArXiv180203426* **1802**, arXiv:1802.03426.

Mirkin, B. L., Clark, S., Zheng, X., Chu, F., White, B. D., Greene, M. and Rebbaa, A. (2005). Identification of midkine as a mediator for intercellular transfer of drug resistance. *Oncogene* **24**, 4965.

Mitsiadis, T. A., Salmivirta, M., Muramatsu, T., Muramatsu, H., Rauvala, H., Lehtonen, E., Jalkanen, M. and Thesleff, I. (1995). Expression of the heparin-binding cytokines, midkine (MK) and HB-GAM (pleiotrophin) is associated with epithelial-mesenchymal interactions during fetal development and organogenesis. *Development* **121**, 37–51.

Miyashiro, M., Kadomatsu, K., Ogata, N., Yamamoto, C., Takahashi, K., Uyama, M., Muramatsu, H. and Muramatsu, T. (1998). Midkine expression in transient retinal ischemia in the rat. *Curr. Eye Res.* **17**, 9–13.

Mohammad, G. and Kowluru, R. A. (2010). Matrix Metalloproteinase-2 in the Development of Diabetic Retinopathy and Mitochondrial Dysfunction. *Lab. Investig. J. Tech. Methods Pathol.* **90**, 1365–1372.

Morin, V., Véron, N. and Marcelle, C. (2017). CRISPR/Cas9 in the Chicken Embryo. In *Avian and Reptilian Developmental Biology: Methods and Protocols* (ed. Sheng, G.), pp. 113–123. New York, NY: Springer New York.

Mulrooney, J., Foley, K., Vineberg, S., Barreuther, M. and Grabel, L. (2000). Phosphorylation of the β1 Integrin Cytoplasmic Domain: Toward an Understanding of Function and Mechanism. *Exp. Cell Res.* **258**, 332–341.

Muramatsu, T. (2002). Midkine and pleiotrophin: two related proteins involved in development, survival, inflammation and tumorigenesis. *J Biochem* **132**, 359–71.

Muramatsu, H., Zou, K., Sakaguchi, N., Ikematsu, S., Sakuma, S. and Muramatsu, T. (2000). LDL Receptor-Related Protein as a Component of the Midkine Receptor. *Biochem. Biophys. Res. Commun.* **270**, 936–941.

Muramatsu, H., Zou, P., Suzuki, H., Oda, Y., Chen, G.-Y., Sakaguchi, N., Sakuma, S., Maeda, N., Noda, M., Takada, Y., et al. (2004). α4β1- and α6β1-integrins are functional receptors for midkine, a heparin-binding growth factor. *J. Cell Sci.* **117**, 5405–5415.

Nagarkatti, P., Pandey, R., Rieder, S. A., Hegde, V. L. and Nagarkatti, M. (2009). Cannabinoids as novel anti-inflammatory drugs. *Future Med. Chem.* **1**, 1333–1349.

Nagase, H. and Woessner, J. F. (1999). Matrix Metalloproteinases. *J. Biol. Chem.* **274**, 21491–21494.

Nagase, H., Visse, R. and Murphy, G. (2006). Structure and function of matrix metalloproteinases and TIMPs. *Cardiovasc. Res.* **69**, 562–573.

Nagashima, M., D'Cruz, T., Hesse, D. and Hitchcock, P. F. (2019a). Midkine-a deficiency causes cell cycle arrest and reactive gliosis in zebrafish Müller glia following photoreceptor cell death. *Invest. Ophthalmol. Vis. Sci.* **60**, 3115–3115.

Nagashima, M., D'Cruz, T. S., Danku, A. E., Hesse, D., Sifuentes, C., Raymond, P. A. and Hitchcock, P. F. (2019b). Midkine-a is required for cell cycle progression of Müller glia glia during neuronal regeneration in the vertebrate retina. *J. Neurosci.*

Nagelhus, E. A., Mathiisen, T. M. and Ottersen, O. P. (2004). Aquaporin-4 in the central nervous system: cellular and subcellular distribution and coexpression with KIR4.1. *Neuroscience* **129**, 905–13.

Naitoh, H., Suganuma, Y., Ueda, Y., Sato, T., Hiramuki, Y., Fujisawa-Sehara, A., Taketani, S. and Araki, M. (2017). Upregulation of matrix metalloproteinase triggers transdifferentiation of retinal pigmented epithelial cells in Xenopus laevis: A Link between inflammatory response and regeneration. *Dev. Neurobiol.* **77**, 1086–1100.

Nakanishi, T., Kadomatsu, K., Okamoto, T., Ichihara-Tanaka, K., Kojima, T., Saito, H., Tomoda, Y. and Muramatsu, T. (1997). Expression of Syndecan-1 and -3 during

Embryogenesis of the Central Nervous System in Relation to Binding with Midkine. *J. Biochem. (Tokyo)* **121**, 197–205.

Nakazawa, T., Shimura, M., Ryu, M., Nishida, K., Pages, G., Pouyssegur, J. and Endo, S. (2008). ERK1 plays a critical protective role against N-methyl-D-aspartate-induced retinal injury. *J Neurosci Res* **86**, 136–44.

Nalli, Y., Dar, M. S., Bano, N., Rasool, J. U., Sarkar, A. R., Banday, J., Bhat, A. Q., Rafia, B., Vishwakarma, R. A., Dar, M. J., et al. (2019). Analyzing the role of cannabinoids as modulators of Wnt/β-catenin signaling pathway for their use in the management of neuropathic pain. *Bioorg. Med. Chem. Lett.* **29**, 1043–1046.

Nelson, C. M., Gorsuch, R. A., Bailey, T. J., Ackerman, K. M., Kassen, S. C. and Hyde, D. R. (2012). Stat3 defines three populations of Muller glia and is required for initiating maximal muller glia proliferation in the regenerating zebrafish retina. *J Comp Neurol* **520**, 4294–311.

Nelson, C. M., Ackerman, K. M., O'Hayer, P., Bailey, T. J., Gorsuch, R. A. and Hyde, D. R. (2013a). Tumor Necrosis Factor-Alpha Is Produced by Dying Retinal Neurons and Is Required for Müller Glia Proliferation during Zebrafish Retinal Regeneration. *J. Neurosci.* **33**, 6524–6539.

Nelson, C. M., Ackerman, K. M., O'Hayer, P., Bailey, T. J., Gorsuch, R. A. and Hyde, D. R. (2013b). Tumor Necrosis Factor-Alpha Is Produced by Dying Retinal Neurons and Is Required for Müller Glia Proliferation during Zebrafish Retinal Regeneration. *J. Neurosci.* **33**, 6524–6539.

Newman, E. A. (2004). Glial modulation of synaptic transmission in the retina. *Glia* **47**, 268–74.

Norrie, J. L., Lupo, M. S., Xu, B., Al Diri, I., Valentine, M., Putnam, D., Griffiths, L., Zhang, J., Johnson, D., Easton, J., et al. (2019). Nucleome Dynamics during Retinal Development. *Neuron* **104**, 512-528.e11.

Nuttall, R. K., Silva, C., Hader, W., Bar-Or, A., Patel, K. D., Edwards, D. R. and Yong, V. W. (2007). Metalloproteinases are enriched in microglia compared with leukocytes and they regulate cytokine levels in activated microglia. *Glia* **55**, 516–526.

Obama, H., Biro, S., Tashiro, T., Tsutsui, J., Ozawa, M., Yoshida, H., Tanaka, H. and Muramatsu, T. (1998). Myocardial infarction induces expression of midkine, a heparin-binding growth factor with reparative activity. *Anticancer Res.* **18**, 145–152.

Ooto, S., Akagi, T., Kageyama, R., Akita, J., Mandai, M., Honda, Y. and Takahashi, M. (2004). Potential for neural regeneration after neurotoxic injury in the adult mammalian retina. *Proc Natl Acad Sci U A* **101**, 13654–9.

Palazuelos, J., Ortega, Z., Díaz-Alonso, J., Guzmán, M. and Galve-Roperh, I. (2012). CB2 Cannabinoid Receptors Promote Neural Progenitor Cell Proliferation via mTORC1 Signaling *. *J. Biol. Chem.* **287**, 1198–1209.

Palazzo, I., Deistler, K., Hoang, T. V., Blackshaw, S. and Fischer, A. J. (2019). NF-κB signaling regulates the formation of proliferating Müller glia-derived progenitor cells in the avian retina. *bioRxiv* 724260.

Palazzo, I., Deistler, K., Hoang, T. V., Blackshaw, S. and Fischer, A. J. (2020a). NF-κB signaling regulates the formation of proliferating Müller glia-derived progenitor cells in the avian retina. *Development*.

Palazzo, I., Deistler, K., Hoang, T. V., Blackshaw, S. and Fischer, A. J. (2020b). NF-κB signaling regulates the formation of proliferating Müller glia-derived progenitor cells in the avian retina. *Development* **147**,.

Pellissier, L. P., Hoek, R. M., Vos, R. M., Aartsen, W. M., Klimczak, R. R., Hoyng, S. A., Flannery, J. G. and Wijnholds, J. (2014). Specific tools for targeting and expression in Müller glial cells. *Mol. Ther. - Methods Clin. Dev.* **1**,.

Penn, J. W., Grobbelaar, A. O. and Rolfe, K. J. (2012). The role of the TGF-β family in wound healing, burns and scarring: a review. *Int. J. Burns Trauma* **2**, 18–28.

Pérez-Martínez, L. and Jaworski, D. M. (2005). Tissue Inhibitor of Metalloproteinase-2 promotes neuronal differentiation by acting as an anti-mitogenic signal. *J. Neurosci. Off. J. Soc. Neurosci.* **25**, 4917–4929.

Pertwee, R. G. (2010). Receptors and Channels Targeted by Synthetic Cannabinoid Receptor Agonists and Antagonists. *Curr. Med. Chem.* **17**, 1360–1381.

Pollak, J., Wilken, M. S., Ueki, Y., Cox, K. E., Sullivan, J. M., Taylor, R. J., Levine, E. M. and Reh, T. A. (2013a). Ascl1 reprograms mouse Muller glia into neurogenic retinal progenitors. *Development* **140**, 2619–2631.

Pollak, J., Wilken, M. S., Ueki, Y., Cox, K. E., Sullivan, J. M., Taylor, R. J., Levine, E. M. and Reh, T. A. (2013b). ASCL1 reprograms mouse Müller glia into neurogenic retinal progenitors. *Dev. Camb. Engl.* **140**, 2619–2631.

Pow, D. V. and Crook, D. K. (1995). Immunocytochemical evidence for the presence of high levels of reduced glutathione in radial glial cells and horizontal cells in the rabbit retina. *Neurosci Lett* **193**, 25–8.

Pow, D. V. and Crook, D. K. (1996). Direct immunocytochemical evidence for the transfer of glutamine from glial cells to neurons: use of specific antibodies directed against the d-stereoisomers of glutamate and glutamine. *Neuroscience* **70**, 295–302.

Powner, M. B., Gillies, M. C., Zhu, M., Vevis, K., Hunyor, A. P. and Fruttiger, M. (2013). Loss of Müller's Cells and Photoreceptors in Macular Telangiectasia Type 2. *Ophthalmology* **120**, 2344–2352.

Qi, M., Ikematsu, S., Maeda, N., Ichihara-Tanaka, K., Sakuma, S., Noda, M., Muramatsu, T. and Kadomatsu, K. (2001). Haptotactic Migration Induced by Midkine INVOLVEMENT OF PROTEIN-TYROSINE PHOSPHATASE ζ, MITOGEN-ACTIVATED PROTEIN KINASE, AND PHOSPHATIDYLINOSITOL 3-KINASE. *J. Biol. Chem.* **276**, 15868–15875.

Qi, J. H., Ebrahem, Q., Yeow, K., Edwards, D. R., Fox, P. L. and Anand-Apte, B. (2002). Expression of Sorsby's Fundus Dystrophy Mutations in Human Retinal Pigment Epithelial Cells Reduces Matrix Metalloproteinase Inhibition and May Promote Angiogenesis. *J. Biol. Chem.* **277**, 13394–13400.

Qiu, X., Hill, A., Packer, J., Lin, D., Ma, Y.-A. and Trapnell, C. (2017a). Single-cell mRNA quantification and differential analysis with Census. *Nat. Methods* **14**, 309–315.

Qiu, X., Mao, Q., Tang, Y., Wang, L., Chawla, R., Pliner, H. A. and Trapnell, C. (2017b). Reversed graph embedding resolves complex single-cell trajectories. *Nat. Methods* **14**, 979–982.

Ramachandran, R., Zhao, X. F. and Goldman, D. (2011). Ascl1a/Dkk/beta-catenin signaling pathway is necessary and glycogen synthase kinase-3beta inhibition is sufficient for zebrafish retina regeneration. *Proc Natl Acad Sci U A* **108**, 15858–63.

Rapino, C., Tortolani, D., Scipioni, L. and Maccarrone, M. (2018). Neuroprotection by (Endo)Cannabinoids in Glaucoma and Retinal Neurodegenerative Diseases. *Curr. Neuropharmacol.* **16**, 959–970.

Raulo, E., Chernousov, M. A., Carey, D. J., Nolo, R. and Rauvala, H. (1994). Isolation of a neuronal cell surface receptor of heparin binding growth-associated molecule (HB-GAM). Identification as N-syndecan (syndecan-3). *J. Biol. Chem.* **269**, 12999–13004.

Raymond, P. A. (1991). Retinal regeneration in teleost fish. *Ciba Found Symp* **160**, 171–86; discussion 186-91.

Reichenbach, A. and Bringmann, A. (2013). New functions of Müller cells. *Glia* **61**, 651–678.

Reiff, T., Huber, L., Kramer, M., Delattre, O., Janoueix-Lerosey, I. and Rohrer, H. (2011). Midkine and Alk signaling in sympathetic neuron proliferation and neuroblastoma predisposition. *Development* **138**, 4699–4708.

Reynolds, P. R., Mucenski, M. L., Cras, T. D. L., Nichols, W. C. and Whitsett, J. A. (2004). Midkine Is Regulated by Hypoxia and Causes Pulmonary Vascular Remodeling. *J. Biol. Chem.* **279**, 37124–37132.

Roger, J., Brajeul, V., Thomasseau, S., Hienola, A., Sahel, J.-A., Guillonneau, X. and Goureau, O. (2006). Involvement of Pleiotrophin in CNTF-mediated differentiation of the late retinal progenitor cells. *Dev. Biol.* **298**, 527–539.

Rompani, S. B. and Cepko, C. L. (2010). A Common Progenitor for Retinal Astrocytes and Oligodendrocytes. *J. Neurosci.* **30**, 4970–4980.

Rosenberg, G. A. (2002). Matrix metalloproteinases in neuroinflammation. *Glia* **39**, 279–291.

Sahay, P., Rao, A., Padhy, D., Sarangi, S., Das, G., Reddy, M. M. and Modak, R. (2017). Functional Activity of Matrix Metalloproteinases 2 and 9 in Tears of Patients With Glaucoma. *Invest. Ophthalmol. Vis. Sci.* **58**, BIO106–BIO113.

Sakaguchi, N., Muramatsu, H., Ichihara-Tanaka, K., Maeda, N., Noda, M., Yamamoto, T., Michikawa, M., Ikematsu, S., Sakuma, S. and Muramatsu, T. (2003). Receptor-type protein tyrosine phosphatase ζ as a component of the signaling receptor complex for midkine-dependent survival of embryonic neurons. *Neurosci. Res.* **45**, 219–224.

Sakakima, H., Kamizono, T., Matsuda, F., Izumo, K., Ijiri, K. and Yoshida, Y. (2006). Midkine and its receptor in regenerating rat skeletal muscle after bupivacaine injection. *Acta Histochem.* **108**, 357–364.

Salama, R. H. M., Muramatsu, H., Zou, P., Okayama, M. and Muramatsu, T. (2006). Midkine, a heparin-binding growth factor, produced by the host enhances metastasis of Lewis lung carcinoma cells. *Cancer Lett.* **233**, 16–20.

Satija, R., Farrell, J. A., Gennert, D., Schier, A. F. and Regev, A. (2015). Spatial reconstruction of single-cell gene expression data. *Nat Biotechnol* **33**, 495–502.

Sato, K. (2015). Effects of Microglia on Neurogenesis. *Glia* **63**, 1394–1405.

Schwitzer, T., Schwan, R., Angioi-Duprez, K., Giersch, A. and Laprevote, V. (2016). The Endocannabinoid System in the Retina: From Physiology to Practical and Therapeutic Applications. *Neural Plast.* **2016**,.

Scott, A. W., Bressler, N. M., Ffolkes, S., Wittenborn, J. S. and Jorkasky, J. (2016). Public Attitudes About Eye and Vision Health. *JAMA Ophthalmol.* **134**, 1111–1118.

Senut, M.-C., Gulati-Leekha, A. and Goldman, D. (2004). An element in the alpha1-tubulin promoter is necessary for retinal expression during optic nerve regeneration but not after eye injury in the adult zebrafish. *J. Neurosci. Off. J. Soc. Neurosci.* **24**, 7663–7673.

Sethi, C. S., Lewis, G. P., Fisher, S. K., Leitner, W. P., Mann, D. L., Luthert, P. J. and Charteris, D. G. (2005). Glial remodeling and neural plasticity in human retinal detachment with proliferative vitreoretinopathy. *Invest Ophthalmol Vis Sci* **46**, 329–42.

Shamsuddin, N. and Kumar, A. (2011). TLR2 mediates the innate response of retinal Muller glia to Staphylococcus aureus. *J Immunol* **186**, 7089–97.

Sharma, P., Gupta, S., Chaudhary, M., Mitra, S., Chawla, B., Khursheed, M. A., Saran, N. K. and Ramachandran, R. (2020). Biphasic Role of Tgf-β Signaling during Müller Glia Reprogramming and Retinal Regeneration in Zebrafish. *iScience* **23**, 100817.

Shen, X., Xi, G., Wai, C. and Clemmons, D. R. (2015). The Coordinate Cellular Response to Insulin-like Growth Factor-I (IGF-I) and Insulin-like Growth Factor-binding Protein-2 (IGFBP-2) Is Regulated through Vimentin Binding to Receptor Tyrosine Phosphatase β (RPTPβ). *J. Biol. Chem.* **290**, 11578–11590.

Shin, D. S., Tokuda, E. Y., Leight, J. L., Miksch, C. E., Brown, T. E. and Anseth, K. S. (2018). Synthesis of Microgel Sensors for Spatial and Temporal Monitoring of Protease Activity. *ACS Biomater. Sci. Eng.* **4**, 378–387.

Sifuentes, C. J., Kim, J.-W., Swaroop, A. and Raymond, P. A. (2016). Rapid, Dynamic Activation of Müller Glial Stem Cell Responses in Zebrafish. *Invest. Ophthalmol. Vis. Sci.* **57**, 5148–5160.

Silva, N. J., Nagashima, M., Li, J., Kakuk-Atkins, L., Ashrafzadeh, M., Hyde, D. R. and Hitchcock, P. F. (2020). Inflammation and matrix metalloproteinase 9 (Mmp-9) regulate photoreceptor regeneration in adult zebrafish. *Glia* **68**, 1445–1465.

Silverman, S. M. and Wong, W. T. (2018a). Microglia in the Retina: Roles in Development, Maturity, and Disease. *Annu. Rev. Vis. Sci.* **4**, 45–77.

Silverman, S. M. and Wong, W. T. (2018b). Microglia in the Retina: Roles in Development, Maturity, and Disease. *Annu. Rev. Vis. Sci.* **4**, 45–77.

Singhal, S., Bhatia, B., Jayaram, H., Becker, S., Jones, M. F., Cottrill, P. B., Khaw, P. T., Salt, T. E. and Limb, G. A. (2012). Human Muller glia with stem cell characteristics differentiate into retinal ganglion cell (RGC) precursors in vitro and partially restore RGC function in vivo following transplantation. *Stem Cells Transl Med* **1**, 188–99.

Slusar, J. E., Cairns, E. A., Szczesniak, A.-M., Bradshaw, H. B., Di Polo, A. and Kelly, M. E. M. (2013). The fatty acid amide hydrolase inhibitor, URB597, promotes retinal ganglion cell neuroprotection in a rat model of optic nerve axotomy. *Neuropharmacology* **72**, 116–125.

Sofroniew, M. V. (2005). Reactive astrocytes in neural repair and protection. *Neuroscientist* **11**, 400–7.

Sofroniew, M. V. (2014). Astrogliosis. *Cold Spring Harb Perspect Biol* **7**, a020420.

Song, J., Zhang, J., Wang, J., Cao, Z., Wang, J., Guo, X. and Dong, W. (2014). β1 integrin modulates tumor growth and apoptosis of human colorectal cancer. *Oncol. Rep.* **32**, 302–308.

Stanchfield, M. L., Webster, S. E., Webster, M. K. and Linn, C. L. (2020). Involvement of HB-EGF/Ascl1/Lin28a Genes in Dedifferentiation of Adult Mammalian Müller Glia. *Front. Mol. Biosci.* **7**,.

Stanke, J., Moose, H. E., El-Hodiri, H. M. and Fischer, A. J. (2010). Comparative study of Pax2 expression in glial cells in the retina and optic nerve of birds and mammals. *J Comp Neurol* **518**, 2316–33.

Stella, N. (2009). Endocannabinoid signaling in microglial cells. *Neuropharmacology* **56**, 244–253.

Stincic, T. L. and Hyson, R. L. (2011). The localization and physiological effects of cannabinoid receptor 1 (CB1) in the brain stem auditory system of the chick. *Neuroscience* **194C**, 150–159.

Stoica, G. E., Kuo, A., Aigner, A., Sunitha, I., Souttou, B., Malerczyk, C., Caughey, D. J., Wen, D., Karavanov, A., Riegel, A. T., et al. (2001). Identification of Anaplastic

Lymphoma Kinase as a Receptor for the Growth Factor Pleiotrophin. *J. Biol. Chem.* **276**, 16772–16779.

Straiker, A. J., Maguire, G., Mackie, K. and Lindsey, J. (1999a). Localization of Cannabinoid CB1 Receptors in the Human Anterior Eye and Retina. *Invest. Ophthalmol. Vis. Sci.* **40**, 2442–2448.

Straiker, A., Stella, N., Piomelli, D., Mackie, K., Karten, H. J. and Maguire, G. (1999b). Cannabinoid CB1 receptors and ligands in vertebrate retina: Localization and function of an endogenous signaling system. *Proc. Natl. Acad. Sci. U. S. A.* **96**, 14565–14570.

Takei, Y., Kadomatsu, K., Matsuo, S., Itoh, H., Nakazawa, K., Kubota, S. and Muramatsu, T. (2001). Antisense Oligodeoxynucleotide Targeted to Midkine, a Heparin-binding Growth Factor, Suppresses Tumorigenicity of Mouse Rectal Carcinoma Cells. *Cancer Res.* **61**, 8486–8491.

Takei, Y., Kadomatsu, K., Goto, T. and Muramatsu, T. (2006). Combinational antitumor effect of siRNA against midkine and paclitaxel on growth of human prostate cancer xenografts. *Cancer* **107**, 864–873.

Takeyama, M., Yoneda, M., Takeuchi, M., Isogai, Z., Ohno-Jinno, A., Kataoka, T., Li, H., Sugita, I., Iwaki, M. and Zako, M. (2010). Increase in matrix metalloproteinase-2 level in the chicken retina after laser photocoagulation. *Lasers Surg. Med.* **42**, 433–441.

Tang, F., Barbacioru, C., Wang, Y., Nordman, E., Lee, C., Xu, N., Wang, X., Bodeau, J., Tuch, B. B., Siddiqui, A., et al. (2009). mRNA-Seq whole-transcriptome analysis of a single cell. *Nat. Methods* **6**, 377–382.

Thillai, K., Lam, H., Sarker, D. and Wells, C. M. (2016). Deciphering the link between PI3K and PAK: An opportunity to target key pathways in pancreatic cancer? *Oncotarget* **8**, 14173–14191.

Todd, L. and Fischer, A. J. (2015). Hedgehog signaling stimulates the formation of proliferating Müller glia-derived progenitor cells in the chick retina. *Dev. Camb. Engl.* **142**, 2610–2622.

Todd, L., Suarez, L., Squires, N., Zelinka, C. P., Gribbins, K. and Fischer, A. J. (2015). Comparative analysis of glucagonergic cells, glia, and the circumferential marginal zone in the reptilian retina. *J. Comp. Neurol.* **524**, 74–89.

Todd, L., Squires, N., Suarez, L. and Fischer, A. J. (2016). Jak/Stat signaling regulates the proliferation and neurogenic potential of Müller glia-derived progenitor cells in the avian retina. *Sci. Rep.* **6**,.

Todd, L., Palazzo, I., Squires, N., Mendonca, N. and Fischer, A. J. (2017). BMP- and TGFbeta-signaling regulate the formation of Muller glia-derived progenitor cells in the avian retina. *Glia*.

Todd, L., Suarez, L., Quinn, C. and Fischer, A. J. (2018). Retinoic Acid-Signaling Regulates the Proliferative and Neurogenic Capacity of Müller Glia-Derived Progenitor Cells in the Avian Retina. *STEM CELLS* **36**, 392–405.

Todd, L., Palazzo, I., Suarez, L., Liu, X., Volkov, L., Hoang, T. V., Campbell, W. A., Blackshaw, S., Quan, N. and Fischer, A. J. (2019). Reactive microglia and IL1β/IL-1R1-signaling mediate neuroprotection in excitotoxin-damaged mouse retina. *J. Neuroinflammation* **16**, 118.

Todd, L., Finkbeiner, C., Wong, C. K., Hooper, M. J. and Reh, T. A. (2020). Microglia Suppress Ascl1-Induced Retinal Regeneration in Mice. *Cell Rep.* **33**, 108507.

Trapnell, C., Roberts, A., Goff, L., Pertea, G., Kim, D., Kelley, D. R., Pimentel, H., Salzberg, S. L., Rinn, J. L. and Pachter, L. (2012). Differential gene and transcript expression analysis of RNA-seq experiments with TopHat and Cufflinks. *Nat Protoc* **7**, 562–78.

Trapnell, C., Cacchiarelli, D., Grimsby, J., Pokharel, P., Li, S., Morse, M., Lennon, N. J., Livak, K. J., Mikkelsen, T. S. and Rinn, J. L. (2014). The dynamics and regulators of cell fate decisions are revealed by pseudotemporal ordering of single cells. *Nat. Biotechnol.* **32**, 381–386.

Tsutsui, J., Uehara, K., Kadomatsu, K., Matsubara, S. and Muramatsu, T. (1991). A new family of heparin-binding factors: Strong conservation of midkine (MK) sequences between the human and the mouse. *Biochem. Biophys. Res. Commun.* **176**, 792–797.

Tsutsui, J., Kadomatsu, K., Matsubara, S., Nakagawara, A., Hamanoue, M., Takao, S., Shimazu, H., Ohi, Y. and Muramatsu, T. (1993). A New Family of Heparin-binding Growth/Differentiation Factors: Increased Midkine Expression in Wilms' Tumor and Other Human Carcinomas. *Cancer Res.* **53**, 1281–1285.

Turner, D. L. and Cepko, C. L. (1987). A common progenitor for neurons and glia persists in rat retina late in development. *Nature* **328**, 131–6.

Ueki, Y. and Reh, T. A. (2013). EGF stimulates Muller glial proliferation via a BMP-dependent mechanism. *Glia* **61**, 778–89.

Ueki, Y., Wilken, M. S., Cox, K. E., Chipman, L., Jorstad, N., Sternhagen, K., Simic, M., Ullom, K., Nakafuku, M. and Reh, T. A. (2015). Transgenic expression of the proneural transcription factor Ascl1 in Müller glia stimulates retinal regeneration in young mice. *Proc. Natl. Acad. Sci.* **112**, 13717–13722.

Ullrich, O., Merker, K., Timm, J. and Tauber, S. (2007). Immune control by endocannabinoids — New mechanisms of neuroprotection? *J. Neuroimmunol.* **184**, 127–135.

Unoki, K., Ohba, N., Arimura, H., Muramatsu, H. and Muramatsu, T. (1994). Rescue of photoreceptors from the damaging effects of constant light by midkine, a retinoic acid-responsive gene product. *Invest. Ophthalmol. Vis. Sci.* **35**, 4063–4068.

Väisänen, A., Kallioinen, M., Dickhoff, K. von, Laatikainen, L., Höyhtyä, M. and Turpeenniemi-Hujanen, T. (1999). Matrix metalloproteinase-2 (MMP-2) immunoreactive protein—a new prognostic marker in uveal melanoma? *J. Pathol.* **188**, 56–62.

Van Rooijen, N. (1989). The liposome-mediated macrophage 'suicide' technique. *J. Immunol. Methods* **124**, 1–6.

Vision impairment and blindness *World Health Organ.*

Wan, J. and Goldman, D. (2016). Retina regeneration in zebrafish. *Curr. Opin. Genet. Dev.* **40**, 41–47.

Wan, J., Ramachandran, R. and Goldman, D. (2012). HB-EGF Is Necessary and Sufficient for Müller Glia Dedifferentiation and Retina Regeneration. *Dev. Cell* **22**, 334–347.

Wan, J., Zhao, X. F., Vojtek, A. and Goldman, D. (2014). Retinal Injury, Growth Factors, and Cytokines Converge on beta-Catenin and pStat3 Signaling to Stimulate Retina Regeneration. *Cell Rep* **9**, 285–97.

Wang, Y. and Navin, N. E. (2015). Advances and Applications of Single Cell Sequencing Technologies. *Mol. Cell* **58**, 598–609.

Wang, Z., Juttermann, R. and Soloway, P. D. (2000). TIMP-2 Is Required for Efficient Activation of proMMP-2 in Vivo. *J. Biol. Chem.* **275**, 26411–26415.

Wang, L.-L., Garcia, C. S., Zhong, X., Ma, S. and Zhang, C.-L. (2020). Rapid and efficient in vivo astrocyte-to-neuron conversion with regional identity and connectivity? *bioRxiv* 2020.08.16.253195.

Webster, N. L. and Crowe, S. M. (2006). Matrix metalloproteinases, their production by monocytes and macrophages and their potential role in HIV-related diseases. *J. Leukoc. Biol.* **80**, 1052–1066.

Welgus, H. G., Jeffrey, J. J., Eisen, A. Z., Roswit, W. T. and Stricklin, G. P. (1985). Human skin fibroblast collagenase: interaction with substrate and inhibitor. *Coll. Relat. Res.* **5**, 167–179.

White, D. T., Sengupta, S., Saxena, M. T., Xu, Q., Hanes, J., Ding, D., Ji, H. and Mumm, J. S. (2017). Immunomodulation-accelerated neuronal regeneration following selective rod photoreceptor cell ablation in the zebrafish retina. *Proc. Natl. Acad. Sci.* **114**, E3719–E3728.

Widera, D., Kaus, A., Kaltschmidt, C. and Kaltschmidt, B. (2008). Neural stem cells, inflammation and NF-κB: basic principle of maintenance and repair or origin of brain tumours? *J. Cell. Mol. Med.* **12**, 459–470.

Wilson, S. W. and Houart, C. (2004). Early steps in the development of the forebrain. *Dev Cell* **6**, 167–81.

Winkler, C. and Yao, S. (2014). The midkine family of growth factors: diverse roles in nervous system formation and maintenance. *Br. J. Pharmacol.* **171**, 905–912.

Wolf, F. A., Angerer, P. and Theis, F. J. (2018). SCANPY: large-scale single-cell gene expression data analysis. *Genome Biol.* **19**, 15.

Xiao, D., Qiu, S., Huang, X., Zhang, R., Lei, Q., Huang, W., Chen, H., Gou, B., Tie, X., Liu, S., et al. (2019). Directed robust generation of functional retinal ganglion cells from Müller glia. *bioRxiv* 735357.

Xu, J.-Y. and Chen, C. (2015). Endocannabinoids in Synaptic Plasticity and Neuroprotection. *Neurosci. Rev. J. Bringing Neurobiol. Neurol. Psychiatry* **21**, 152–168.

Xu, C., Zhu, S., Wu, M., Han, W. and Yu, Y. (2014). Functional Receptors and Intracellular Signal Pathways of Midkine (MK) and Pleiotrophin (PTN). *Biol. Pharm. Bull.* **37**, 511–520.

Yamada, T., Yoshiyama, Y., Sato, H., Seiki, M., Shinagawa, A. and Takahashi, M. (1995). White matter microglia produce membrane-type matrix metalloprotease, an activator of gelatinase A, in human brain tissues. *Acta Neuropathol. (Berl.)* **90**, 421–424.

Yamagata, M., Yan, W. and Sanes, J. R. (2021). A cell atlas of the chick retina based on single-cell transcriptomics. *eLife* **10**, e63907.

Yang, W., Li, Q., Wang, S.-Y., Gao, F., Qian, W.-J., Li, F., Ji, M., Sun, X.-H., Miao, Y. and Wang, Z. (2016). Cannabinoid receptor agonists modulate calcium channels in rat retinal müller cells. *Neuroscience* **313**, 213–224.

Yao, K., Qiu, S., Tian, L., Snider, W. D., Flannery, J. G., Schaffer, D. V. and Chen, B. (2016). Wnt Regulates Proliferation and Neurogenic Potential of Muller Glial Cells via a Lin28/let-7 miRNA-Dependent Pathway in Adult Mammalian Retinas. *Cell Rep* **17**, 165–78.

Yao, K., Qiu, S., Wang, Y. V., Park, S. J. H., Mohns, E. J., Mehta, B., Liu, X., Chang, B., Zenisek, D., Crair, M. C., et al. (2018). Restoration of vision after de novo genesis of rod photoreceptors in mammalian retinas. *Nature* **560**, 484–488.

Yazulla, S., Studholme, K. M., McINTOSH, H. H. and Fan, S.-F. (2000). Cannabinoid receptors on goldfish retinal bipolar cells: Electron-microscope immunocytochemistry and whole-cell recordings. *Vis. Neurosci.* **17**, 391–401.

Zelinka, C. P., Scott, M. A., Volkov, L. and Fischer, A. J. (2012). The Reactivity, Distribution and Abundance of Non-Astrocytic Inner Retinal Glial (NIRG) Cells Are Regulated by Microglia, Acute Damage, and IGF1. *PLOS ONE* **7**, e44477.

Zelinka, C. P., Volkov, L., Goodman, Z. A., Todd, L., Palazzo, I., Bishop, W. A. and Fischer, A. J. (2016). mTor signaling is required for the formation of proliferating Müller glia-derived progenitor cells in the chick retina. *Dev. Camb. Engl.* **143**, 1859–1873.

Zhang, J., Bai, S., Zhang, X., Nagase, H. and Sarras, M. P. (2003). The expression of gelatinase A (MMP-2) is required for normal development of zebrafish embryos. *Dev. Genes Evol.* **213**, 456–463.

Zhao, H., Bernardo, M. M., Osenkowski, P., Sohail, A., Pei, D., Nagase, H., Kashiwagi, M., Soloway, P. D., DeClerck, Y. A. and Fridman, R. (2004). Differential Inhibition of Membrane Type 3 (MT3)-Matrix Metalloproteinase (MMP) and MT1-MMP by Tissue Inhibitor of Metalloproteinase (TIMP)-2 and TIMP-3 Regulates Pro-MMP-2 Activation. *J. Biol. Chem.* **279**, 8592–8601.

Zhao, X.-F., Wan, J., Powell, C., Ramachandran, R., Myers, M. G. and Goldman, D. (2014a). Leptin and IL-6 family cytokines synergize to stimulate Müller glia reprogramming and retina regeneration. *Cell Rep.* **9**, 272–284.

Zhao, X. F., Wan, J., Powell, C., Ramachandran, R., Myers, M. G., Jr. and Goldman, D. (2014b). Leptin and IL-6 family cytokines synergize to stimulate muller glia reprogramming and retina regeneration. *Cell Rep* **9**, 272–84.

Zhou, Z. Y., Packialakshmi, B., Makkar, S. K., Dridi, S. and Rath, N. C. (2014). Effect of butyrate on immune response of a chicken macrophage cell line. *Vet. Immunol. Immunopathol.* **162**, 24–32.

Zhou, H., Su, J., Hu, X., Zhou, C., Li, H., Chen, Z., Xiao, Q., Wang, B., Wu, W., Sun, Y., et al. (2020). Glia-to-Neuron Conversion by CRISPR-CasRx Alleviates Symptoms of Neurological Disease in Mice. *Cell* **181**, 590-603.e16.

Zibetti, C., Liu, S., Wan, J., Qian, J. and Blackshaw, S. (2019). Epigenomic profiling of retinal progenitors reveals LHX2 is required for developmental regulation of open chromatin. *Commun. Biol.* **2**,.

Zou, K., Muramatsu, H., Ikematsu, S., Sakuma, S., Salama, R. H. M., Shinomura, T., Kimata, K. and Muramatsu, T. (2000). A heparin-binding growth factor, midkine, binds to a chondroitin sulfate proteoglycan, PG-M/versican. *Eur. J. Biochem.* **267**, 4046–4053.

Zuber, M. E., Gestri, G., Viczian, A. S., Barsacchi, G. and Harris, W. A. (2003). Specification of the vertebrate eye by a network of eye field transcription factors. *Development* **130**, 5155–67.

Zucker, S., Drews, M., Conner, C., Foda, H. D., DeClerck, Y. A., Langley, K. E., Bahou, W. F., Docherty, A. J. P. and Cao, J. (1998). Tissue Inhibitor of Metalloproteinase-2 (TIMP-2) Binds to the Catalytic Domain of the Cell Surface Receptor, Membrane Type 1-Matrix Metalloproteinase 1 (MT1-MMP). *J. Biol. Chem.* **273**, 1216–1222.